Dramatizing Dementia

Dramatizing Dementia:
Madness in the Plays
of Tennessee Williams

Jacqueline O'Connor

Bowling Green State University Popular Press
Bowling Green, OH 43403

Permission to quote from manuscript material in the Harry Ransom Humanities Research Center at the University of Texas at Austin is gratefully acknowledged.

Library of Congress Cataloging-in-Publication Data
O'Connor, Jacqueline.
    Dramatizing dementia : madness in the plays of Tennessee Williams / Jacqueline O'Connor.
        p.   cm.
    Includes bibliographical references (p.   ) and index.
    ISBN 0-87972-741-1 (cloth). -- 0-87972-742-X (pbk.)
    1. Williams, Tennessee, 1911-1983--Characters--Mentally ill.
2. Williams, Tennessee, 1911-1983--Knowledge --Psychology.
3. Literature and mental illness--Southern States. 4. Mental illness in literature. 5. Drama--Psychological aspects. 6. Mentally ill in literature. I. Title.
PS3545.I5365Z795   1997
812'.54--dc21   97-20537
                                                                      CIP

Cover design by Dumm Art

Contents

Acknowledgments

Many people supported this project, and without them it would not have been completed. Ruby Cohn generously offered her expertise throughout the book's preparation. Sherman Randleas saw me through all the beginning stages of preparing the manuscript. Generous financial assistance from the University of California at Davis and Stephen F. Austin State University allowed me some essential research opportunities. The library staff of the Harry Ransom Center at the University of Texas were very helpful in providing necessary research materials for my use; Pat Fox was particularly obliging. The editors at Bowling Green State University Popular Press, especially Pat Browne and Barbara Solosy, were patient and supportive during the publication process. Finally, I would like to thank my family for their love and their acceptance of me, especially my father, John O'Connor.

Preface

This book began from an interest in literary representations of madness, especially dramatic representations. My original impulse was to explore the topic in the works of a number of American playwrights, for in reading and viewing modern American plays, I had seen in many of them madness as both a theme and a character motivation. I became particularly interested in dramatic works in which a character's instability or unconventional behavior resulted in institutionalization, or works in which the mental institution itself was the play's setting, usually acting as a metaphor for a loss of freedom or control. My reading led me to *A Streetcar Named Desire,* a play that dramatizes just such a loss of freedom. Blanche's departure at the conclusion of the drama, accompanied by state hospital staff and threatened with a straitjacket, epitomizes the dangers that mental instability poses for the unprotected. Further exploration of Williams's drama convinced me that his plays alone might form the basis of study for my book: from the beginning to the end of his long career as a dramatist, he created characters and situations that touched on this theme.

The dementia of my title is not clinical. Rather than attempting to psychoanalyze the characters, as others with more expertise have done, I have used the social situations within the dramas themselves to define the terms of my argument. Literary madness shares with literal madness one terrifying similarity; it is often defined by comparing the behavior of one suspected of madness with those around them. For that reason it is not surprising that dramatic representations of madness often reflect and deflect the question of sanity onto the play's world: Shakespeare knew this when he wrote *King Lear.*

My approach to the material grew naturally out of the material itself, as clear patterns began to form early in my research. As a result, I have organized my analysis of the plays according to several recurring themes: confinement, women, language, artists. In many ways, these were major concerns of Williams in all his work, so that the intersection of these topics with the more pervasive topic of madness is not surprising. Other critics have demonstrated the ubiquity of the topic in Williams's oeuvre, but this book is unique in its total devotion to the subject.

vii

The dramas that play major roles in my discussion are as follows: *Portrait of a Madonna, The Glass Menagerie, A Streetcar Named Desire, Suddenly Last Summer, The Night of the Iguana, The Two-Character Play,* and *Clothes for a Summer Hotel.* They represent the full range of Williams's stylistic development, and mark a variety of points in his forty-year career. Some of these plays number among the best-known of all American dramas, while others are familiar only to scholars and theater practitioners. Since my organization is thematic, some plays are discussed more than once in different contexts, for my intention is to move beyond separate analysis of individual plays to demonstrate the ways that Williams established connections among important social and artistic concerns by dramatizing them through a common lens.

While my study is indebted to a wide range of texts that treat madness as a philosophical, psychological, social, or literary issue, the bulk of my discussion concentrates on the play texts and appropriate biographical materials. While I have attempted to move beyond a long-standing approach to Williams that analyzes his life along with his work, I have discovered that a total separation of the two is impossible. As much as any modern writer, and more than most, Williams's life seems to have been a collection of interlocking and sometimes contradictory fictions; the same could be said of his characters, so they can be analytically useful to examine the free interplay he seems to have encouraged between one kind of fiction and the other. Perhaps, then, this book will also provide some small insight into Williams's fear of and fascination with madness.

1

Binding Ties: Introduction

Oh Laura, Laura, I tried to leave you behind me,
but I am more faithful than I intended to be.
          —Tom in *The Glass Menagerie*

She is a metal forged by love
too volatile, too fiery thin
so that her substance will be lost
as sudden lightning or as wind.
          —from "Elegy for Rose" by Tennessee Williams

On a postcard to his grandparents dated October 1939, soon after his arrival in New York, Tennessee Williams writes that the play season has just begun. Commenting on his own place in the theater world, he says: "I am meeting everybody and beginning to feel important because of the sudden attention they give me. They look at me like I was a goose about to lay a dozen golden eggs!"[1] During his long career, Williams did indeed produce some golden eggs, among them *The Glass Menagerie*, which won the Drama Critics' Circle Award in 1945. Williams won both the Drama Critics' Circle Award and the Pulitzer Prize for *A Streetcar Named Desire* in 1948; he was awarded both once more for *Cat on a Hot Tin Roof* in 1955, and the Drama Critics' Circle Award for *The Night of the Iguana* in 1962. But the awards barely begin to describe his status in the theatrical world from *The Glass Menagerie* to his death in 1983. His attitude about fame may be summed up by these words from a letter to his mother, dated March 21, 1939, written to inform her that he had won the Group Theatre prize: "For every bouquet in writing you get ten kicks in the face—which prevents one from feeling too elated over an occasional honor."[2]

The sheer volume of the artistic work Williams produced in his lifetime rivals that of most writers; he is considered one of the greatest American playwrights. Much of his later work is judged inferior to his masterpieces of the 1940s and 1950s, when he dominated Broadway, but he continued to write, rewrite, and arrange productions long after he was convinced that the critics had turned against him.

2 Dramatizing Dementia

Born in Mississippi on March 26, 1911, Thomas Lanier Williams began writing while still a boy, and had his entry into an essay contest published in the national magazine *Smart Set* when he was sixteen. A year later, his short story "The Vengeance of Nitocris" was accepted by *Weird Tales*. His biographer, Donald Spoto, calls the story "suprisingly lurid," noting that despite its schoolboy prose, the tale's shocking ending foreshadowed much of Williams's later work (27). Other documents from this period attest to his developing style: letters to his parents, written from Europe while on a trip with his grandfather, show his predilection for flowery speech. He describes the bed at the Biltmore Hotel in New York upon their return from the continent as "seductive as Paradise to the damned." In another letter he exposes his preoccupation with confinement, which becomes a central theme in his work; when writing from Montreux after a visit to the nearby Castle of Chillon, he insists that if "captivity for life were imposed upon me, I should prefer the Castle of Chillon to any other prison."[3]

While working in St. Louis in the factory where his father was employed, he became involved with small local theatrical groups that staged several of his plays. The Mummers produced the full-length *Candles to the Sun* in 1937. After attending the University of Missouri at Columbia, and Washington University in St. Louis, he received his bachelor's degree in English, from the University of Iowa, in 1938. His letters to his mother from college attest to his wit, and foreshadow the understated humor in even his grimmest plays. Having flunked R.O.T.C. at the University of Missouri, a great shame to his father, he writes from Iowa a few years later about landing a role in a student production of Shakespeare: "I am enlisted as a soldier in King Henry IV's army—next major play—fortunately they did not know about my record in the R.O.T.C."[4]

After graduation, he began a life of wandering; although he worked at a variety of jobs over the next six years, his energy went into his writing. Upon winning a special honorable mention from a Group Theatre contest for his collection of one-act plays, *American Blues,* Williams caught the attention of agent Audrey Wood; so in 1939 he began one of the important professional relationships of his career. Her agency, Liebling-Wood, represented Williams from that time until 1971. In the early years Wood relentlessly pursued success for him, and demonstrated belief in his future. In a letter that she wrote him about the difficulty selling his story "Portrait of a Girl in Glass," she insisted that one day "I shall be full of glee when all of Williams is sold in book form and people rush by the thousands to read it. I shall gurgle and make other noises and people will think I've gone mad but I think you will understand."[5] He changed his name at this time: the short story "The Field of Blue Children" was his first published work to list its author as Tennessee Williams.

During his college days, indications begin to appear in his correspondence of the emotional problems of his older sister, Rose. She writes to him from Knoxville in 1937: "I know that you were all glad to ship me down here. My spirits are low this afternoon." She adds that her aunt "seems to accomplish so much that I feel like crawling into a hole and never reappearing."[6] During that year, Rose saw a number of psychologists, was briefly hospitalized, and then released, from the Farmington state asylum (Spoto 63). Williams's transfer to the University of Iowa took him away from home in the fall, so he was absent when Rose's doctors convinced her parents that a prefrontal lobotomy was the only possibility for cure. Williams blamed his mother, who in turn claimed that her husband, Cornelius, made the final decision. Clearly, however, the family shared the burden for what happened to Rose, and no matter what he said, Williams would seek many times to exorcise his guilt over Rose's illness. Rose imagery recurs throughout his plays, and the details of his sister's confinement and treatment frequently appear in the dramas about madness that form the focus of this study.

In another letter dated July 8, 1943, with a return address of the "State Hospital, Farmington, Missouri," Rose writes to Tennessee of "trying not to die," and of her conviction that he would love her even if she murdered someone. If she dies, she wishes to be cremated, her ashes mixed with his. This is one of a group of four letters from Rose to Tennessee over the course of twenty years, testifying to the changing condition of Rose's mind; this final one expresses the despair that overtakes her after her permanent institutionalization. The letters, filed together in the archives at the Humanities Research Center in Austin, chronicle the loss of a vibrant life to the ravages of mental illness. The childish scrawl of the earliest one, dated 1922, when Rose is in Mississippi, visiting her grandparents, testifies to her still carefree life. The next, written in 1926, places Rose at All Saints College, sounding grownup and immersed in the social scene. The one from Knoxville on the first day of the year of the lobotomy speaks of her growing depression, despite her still active life. The letter of 1943 indicates Rose's withdrawal from the concerns of the living, her interests shifting to the inevitability of her death.

Other Williams family documents indicate Rose's retreat from the affairs of the world. Among the vast collection of Williams papers and typescripts housed at the University of Texas, seven scrapbooks compiled by his mother, Edwina, mark the events of Tennessee's long career. While the playwright's accomplishments are the spotlight, mementoes of his brother, Dakin; his grandfather, Walter Dakin; and Edwina help fill the pages. No mention of Rose is made, testifying to her lack of place in the family records. Tennessee's father, Cornelius, is also curiously absent from the scrapbooks' documentation; this absence attests to the emotional distance between Cornelius and Edwina.

Much has been written about the Williams family: the parents' incompatibility, their "failure" to handle Rose, Dakin's part in Williams's confinement in 1969; however, the familial relations were not always strained, and all members of the family showed support for Tennessee during his early years of professional struggle. His mother's letters are a poignant mixture of maternal concern, a take-charge managerial quality, and unquestionable loyalty and support. She constantly cautions him to save his money, as she says, for "that proverbial 'rainy day.'" She sounds a good deal like Amanda Wingfield, in her admonishments to Williams to prepare for the future, lest it become "everlasting regret."

In a letter to his mother written in May of 1943, Tennessee objects to the plans that Edwina is making for Rose, and asks that his mother not place her back in the asylum: "That, I am sure, would be the final blow, as she would almost certainly give up all hope if her limited freedom that she has with Mrs. Turner is taken away."[7] Williams felt that he and Rose were similar in emotional makeup, that as early as his teens he exhibited signs of neurosis. He notes in his *Memoirs* that at the age of sixteen "my deep nervous problems approached what might well have been a crisis as shattering as that which broke my sister's mind, lastingly, when she was in her twenties" (16). A summer trip to Europe with his grandfather seems to have calmed young Tom's nerves, but he was correct in fearing confinement for his sister.

In 1969, after years of daily alcohol and drug use, Tennessee Williams demonstrated a weakened mental condition that alarmed those closest to him. Concerned friends called his brother to Key West, hoping Dakin could convince Tennessee to receive treatment. Dakin persuaded him to return with him to St. Louis, in order to seek help at Barnes Hospital, where Rose had been treated during the 1930s in the early days of her illness. Williams voluntarily had himself committed to Barnes, where he was confined in the psychiatric division for a period of three months. After his release, he entered a time of increased productivity, and over the last twelve years of his life he managed to maintain some control over his drinking and drug use. The short confinement may have prolonged his life, for it allowed him to curb the narcotics abuse that threatened to destroy him. Thereafter, however, he lived with the knowledge that he was correct in fearing that Rose's fate might become his own. As Spoto comments, up until 1969, he "had been somehow able to avoid the extreme to which Rose (and Blanche DuBois, Catharine Holly, and others in his plays) had been subjected—unwilling confinement in an asylum. . . . What must never happen, happened" (316).

The material available on the personal life of the playwright is extensive. Accounts of his life have been recorded by family and friends. Not only did Williams publish his own memoirs, but his mother and brother both wrote books about him from their viewpoints. According to the playwright himself, he drew from his personal experience to create his drama; he looked to Hart Crane as a model, and it was Crane's "insistence on transmuting the raw material of one's own life into the stuff of poetry and drama, that stung Tom Williams as perhaps the single great challenge he was facing, then or thereafter" (Spoto 59).

Spoto also tells us that Williams wrote to Audrey Wood in 1942 about the biggest threat to his integrity as a writer, "the temptation to take the easy way out by not dealing with the things he knew best—family pain, mental instability, emotional obsessions, the conflict between the love of solitude and the desire for human comfort" (Spoto 103). Luckily for the multitudes who have enjoyed his plays, both as texts and as performances, he did not choose this way, but faced his obsessions and conflicts. He also writes to Audrey Wood in a letter dated December 1939 that he has "only one major theme for all my work which is the destructive impact of society on the sensitive, non-conformist individual."[8] That sensitive individual was often subject to nervous disorders, and frequently the experiences of his sister found their way into his plays.

Williams writes convincingly about the kind of life a patient faced in the institution. Besides his own experience with Rose, his lover Frank Merlo had a nephew who was treated in 1952 at the New Jersey state sanitarium for a "mild form of dementia praecox." Williams reports in a letter to the Rev. Dakin that the young man and Frank "grew up as brothers so Frank is very disturbed over this and has to spend a great deal of time visiting him. The nephew is now taking insulin shock treatments."[9] Williams's familiarity with treatment and care of the insane came, therefore, not only from his own family experience, but from his witnessing Frank's family situation. This might have convinced Williams that his was not a unique experience, and that although many people do not speak of it, most have some experience with madness, if not personally, then through a family member or friend.

Williams's closeness to his sister, and his commitment to writing about what he knew best, enabled him to write of madness without flinching. He did not include mad characters in his plays merely because they are a part of a long literary tradition (although they are); he included them because he knew them. Those who experience madness personally, or who observe it in a close family member or friend, cannot afford the luxury of ignoring it. They must find a way to meet it, to acknowledge it, to live with it. Williams found his way through his drama. It was because of Rose that he wrote so often about insanity: not merely because he was obsessed with her madness, but because her madness strongly suggested that his lurked around the corner, and that somehow he must evade it, outrun it, keep it from conquering him. His interest in the sensitive individual destroyed by society found an appropriate vehicle in the subject of madness: the ravaged mind results from the brutality and destructive nature of the society.

The mad characters he created seek acceptance, love, and fulfillment; their actions and words press against the limits of acceptable behavior, but their predicament never strays from distinctly human concerns. Although the characters in his plays are unusual people, they are not unknown to us; they are like ourselves or our family members or our friends. Even though they speak rhythmically, their fears are our fears, their weaknesses our weaknesses. Williams's unique brand of theater may be better known for the violence, the perversity, the deviance of the worlds he creates; if these, however, were his only outstanding qualities, he would by now be forgotten, for the art of today's world has far surpassed in violence, perversity, and deviance what Williams presented in his time. Nor are his plays now appreciated merely for their historical value, for the view they provide of postwar America and beyond. Some of his plays are dated, but his finest works endure. A handful of the best plays focus on madness, for it is a subject never far from the author's mind.

Even though I cannot ignore Williams's family history for its part in directing him to this theme, what I want to explore in this work is the way his writings about insanity contributed to his unique vision of humanity. In a journal written in 1949, he writes of his own mental condition, and of a period "full of the dullness and tedium of a mind that no longer particularly cares for existence. Yet is desperate to continue, to survive, to fight the way through a mind that fears breaking because of its constant neurosis. But must not and will *not*." His most memorable characters display a propensity for neurosis, as well as a desperate need to survive. A *Time* article on Williams dated March 9, 1962, called him the "nightmare merchant of Broadway," a playwright with a dark, narrow vision of life whose "special compassion is for the 'people who are not meant to win,' the lost, the odd, the strange, the difficult people—fragile spirits, who lack talons for the jungle."[10] It is to those odd, fragile spirits that I direct my attention.

"Madness," Lillian Feder writes, "is currently used to describe a wide variety of contradictory attitudes and almost any conduct that can either be justified or attacked as extreme" (xi). A brief discussion of some of the modern theories of madness will show the range of thought on the topic, demonstrating that while a comprehensive definition of madness is not possible, common perspectives do exist.

R. D. Laing attempts in *The Divided Self* to "make madness, and the process of going mad, comprehensible," calling his work a study in "existential psychology and psychiatry" (9). In Laing's view, the schizoid person cannot be discussed without some acknowledgment of that person's place in the world, or, more precisely, the degree to which the person feels isolated or out of touch with the world. Laing's book was published within a year of another work on madness, Foucault's *Madness and Civilization*.[11] One aspect that the works share is an emphasis on society's participation in the making of mental patients: although Laing and others in the mental health field admit to the existence of the schizophrenic individual, a good part of this diagnosis depends on the individual's relationship to others, as well as on the reactions of others to the individual's behavior. In *The Order of Things*, Foucault takes this assertion further to argue:

The history of madness would be the history of the Other—of that which, for a given culture, is at once interior and foreign, therefore to be excluded (so as to exorcise the internal danger) but by being shut away (in order to reduce its otherness). (*Order* xxiv)

What Foucault suggests, therefore, is that madness consists of a strangeness that we all share: by identifying and isolating its existence in others, we can relieve ourselves of the fear that this strangeness is our own. If Foucault is correct, this may account for the ubiquitous appearance of madness in literature, which hinges on the creation of fictional persons who can bear the burden of strangeness for us, while we see them as Other. In some sense, the strangeness is "shut away" in the work of literature, for the madness exists in a fictional form that offers no danger to the reader, except to the degree that the writer manipulates the reader's association with the mad characters.

Besides the sociological approach to madness, a medical model for mental illness dominates contemporary approaches. Theories of the neurological origins of madness, such as the fairly recent supposition that schizophrenia results from a chemical imbalance in the brain, have directed clinical inquiries towards physiological explanations of mental illness; such approaches provide little insight to the mad characters of a literary work, and my study will not attempt to make such diagnoses. A study of madness differs from a study of madness in literature, and as Feder claims,

Although the mad characters or personae of literature may be modeled on actual persons or the authors themselves, it is also true that literary constructs of the extreme possibilities of mental experience differ in important respects from actual manifestations of madness. (xiii)

One such difference must be in the inability of the literary critic to make a physiological diagnosis of the characters. This is especially true in a work of drama, when the characters are known to the audience primarily by what they do and say, not by narrative commentary that may make substantial contributions in a novel to the reader's understanding of the motivations and mental condition of its characters.

In my exploration of this subject, I will use certain words interchangeably to describe the behavior of characters included in my study: madness, insanity, mental illness. Thomas Szasz, a psychiatrist who wrote "The Myth of Mental Illness," protested the association of illness with what he calls problems of living:

The assumption is made that some neurological defect, perhaps a very subtle one, will ultimately be found to explain all the disorders of thinking and behavior . . . which implies that people's troubles cannot be caused by conflicting personal needs, opinions, social aspirations, values and so forth. (*Ideology* 13)

From a medical viewpoint Szasz may be correct in assuming that the term "mental illness" implies neurological illness, but in ordinary use it describes behavior that the lay person would not distinguish from "madness." Szasz insists that "we call people mentally ill when their personal conduct violates certain ethical, political, and social norms" (*Law* 17). Such a broad definition, according to Szasz, allows for a wide variety of unusual behavior to be categorized as mental illness: "This explains why many historical figures, from Jesus to Castro, and from Job to Hitler, have been diagnosed as suffering from this or that psychiatric malady" (17).

Szasz's definition, linked as it is to both personal conduct and social norms, summarizes the kind of approach that my study takes to Williams's plays. While such a sociological approach to madness is but one of a variety of viewpoints, it seems to me to be the most appropriate approach to an examination of Williams's mad people. My character analyses will include theories of Foucault, Szasz, and others, where they seem to me illuminating. Although Williams had an awareness of clinical practices and diagnoses, his plays present madness as behavior deemed unfit or unacceptable to the society of the play. This ranges from nervousness to lying, from excessive drinking to promiscuous sexual behavior. The vagueness of the definition is one of its most significant qualities; if madness is loosely defined, its meaning subject to shifting perspectives, all forms of unusual behavior might be included. William Kleb, in a recent article on Foucault and *A Streetcar Named Desire,* quotes Eric Bentley on this issue: "Can a sister just send someone to an asylum without any medical advice? If so, which of us is safe?" (Kleb 39). Williams's plays suggest that none of us are.

Inherited insanity, presupposing genetic tendencies towards madness, is suggested in a few of the plays, for Felice and Clare of *The Two-Character Play* refer often to their insane father; similarly, Alma's nervous problems in *Summer and Smoke* might result from inheriting her mother's genes, rather than from her anxieties about her mother's odd behavior. As William Kleb points out, we might consider the implications of genetic insanity in *Streetcar:* "Blanche stands for Stella's psychological inheritance: a threat not only to her marriage but to the baby in her womb" (Kleb 32). But the madness results most frequently from personal circumstances and social pressures. Despite the nature of my subject matter, and its connection to the fields of psychiatry and medicine, this remains a literary study; my interest lies in the personal and social positions of the mad characters in these plays, as well as in the statements the plays make about the role of the outsider.

Williams presents madness variously: a character embraces illusion to the extent of inhibiting that individual's ability to survive; a character exhibits extreme nervousness, and hypersensitivity so pronounced as to severely restrict or prevent communication with others; a character insists on relating incidents or theories so unacceptable to the other characters in the play that the possibility of the truth of these stories promotes fear and denial within the community. Although the audience may know the story is true, the characters may doubt the story, insisting that the teller is mad.[12] The last characteristic differs from the first two in that it hinges on the perception of the mad person by other characters in the play, whereas the first two rely primarily on character development.

The term madness may seem strong for the symptoms I have listed above, and yet each qualifies as the sort of behavior that threatens the freedom of the character who embraces it. If a character is confined in a mental institution, then that character fits the definition of the insane, according to the society of the play.[13] In his study of the career of the mental patient, Erving Goffman notes that the psychiatric view of a person becomes significant only in so far as this view itself alters his social fate—an alteration which seems to become fundamental in our society *when, and only when, the person is put through the process of hospitalization* [my emphasis]. (128)

Goffman goes on to argue that despite the varieties in kind or degree of mental illness, institutionalization usually brings out a common character in this diverse group, a "tribute to the power of social forces" (129).

One striking characteristic of all the mad characters is their inability to control their impulses, usually self-destructive, and in some cases, sexual.[14] In a study titled *Difference and Pathology*, Sander Gilman claims that of all models of pathology, "one of the most powerful is mental illness. For the most elementally frightening possibility is loss of control over the self" (23). And from Goffman: "This view [losing control] of oneself would seem to be one of the most pervasively threatening things that can happen to the self in our society" (131). The mentally ill become the Other because they cannot be the self, for the "mad are perceived as the antithesis to the control and reason that define the self" (*Difference* 23). Gilman, like Foucault, sees the projection of unreasonableness onto others as self-deceptive:

within everyone's fantasy life there exists a play of aggression not essentially different from that of the initial moment of individuation, an incipient madness that we control with more or less success. (*Difference* 23)

This view of the mad person as a creation of society, an obvious outcome of the repression and fear of difference, of personal conduct that deviates from the norm, pervades the writings of Szasz and Gilman, who see madness as a social construction. Neither denies that emotional problems exist, but that in speaking of madness, we must recognize that our categorizing of the mad cannot be completely separated from our need to define ourselves as normal.

Establishing that the behavior of the insane deviates from the norm leads to a problem that confronts any theorist who seeks to define or explore madness: how to study the mad without speaking of them as the Other? Shoshana Felman, in her study of *Writing and Madness*, states this as Foucault's implicit question in *Madness and Civilization:*

how can we comprehend without objectifying, without excluding? . . . [H]ow can we comprehend without enclosing in ourselves, without confining? How can we understand the Subject, without transforming him (or her) into an object? (41-42)

These are questions that encompass far more than the discussion of madness, and relate to the most fundamental issues that confront everyone who studies the behavior of a group; as Foucault and even Felman acknowledge by the publications of their books, these questions should not halt the inquiry itself. They should, however, prompt the writer to acknowledge this dilemma at the outset. Sander Gilman explores the use of stereotypes in his book *Difference and Pathology*, and maintains: "Stereotypes are a crude set of mental representations of the world. . . . They perpetuate a needed sense of difference between the 'self' and the 'object,' which becomes the 'Other'" (17-18). He accepts the formation of stereotypes, even as he sets about to undermine their power; he examines their origin and structure:

Stereotypes arise when self-integration is threatened. They are therefore part of our way of dealing with the instabilities of our perception of the world. This is not to say that they are good, only that they are necessary. (18)

An acknowledgment that the category of the mad exists is essential to my study, but I struggle to avoid the objectification that permeates American society's view of the mad. I will seek to temper any tendencies toward objectification by emphasizing the universal traits of the characters, what Williams himself accomplishes successfully. Even when presenting grotesque figures, he manages to convey their humanity, preventing us from completely denying their place in our midst.

In embarking on a discussion of the mad characters in drama, I must highlight another consideration: when presenting madness onstage the dramatist has different constraints than does the novelist. The playwright is denied the luxury of narrative in which to explain the character's mental disposition. In performance, we see and hear the madness when experiencing the play, although when reading the play we may get some assistance from stage directions. If the playwright wishes to engage audience sympathies with the mad person, then the presentation of madness must include, not alienate. This might be one of Williams's greatest accomplishments in presenting the mad person to his viewers and readers: as William Kleb argues in his recent article on Williams and Foucault, Blanche, alone in the kitchen in scene one, "gathers our gaze and we begin to see the world through her eyes. From then on, no matter how her difference is defined and displayed, something of this point of view remains" (40). This may be especially true of Blanche, but it holds true for other Williams characters.

Williams's mad characters are usually women who cling to illusions, and, as one reviewer described Blanche: "[I]magine a woman who lives so corruptly in a world of illusion that the merest breath of reality makes her hysterical" (Whitworth 17). Williams's women are often sexually promiscuous, while at the same time exhibiting a streak of prudishness that conflicts with their desire for intimate companionship. The description of one of the few men who belong to the group of mad characters, the Reverend T. Shannon of *The Night of the Iguana,* shows how these same qualities clash and often promote mental collapse; Shannon is described thus:

a man of great charm and some madness . . . a man of irreconcilable elements in his nature. A Puritan with a sexuality that he spends his life, his nerves, in a violent but unsuccessful effort to hold in check. He has cracked up twice: A third time is imminent it seems.[15]

This description echoes Williams's assessment of his own character: a mixture of the Puritan and Cavalier strains, or as Nancy Tischler quotes him: "I'm a rebellious Puritan" (*Rebellious Puritan* 16). In attributing such a mixture to Shannon, Williams emphasizes the effect this conflict has on the sanity of the individual.

This version of *Iguana* has Shannon saying something else about himself which provides insight into the type of person who suffers from emotional breakdowns. When Hannah comments on his kindness, he laughingly replies: "When I'm not too absorbed in problems of my own, I can feel other people's. It's good medicine for me, therapy for me. To feel other people's problems and get my mind for just a little while off my own."[16] Most of the characters who succumb to madness are totally self-absorbed. This often makes them unbearable to those around them; since they are incapable of showing empathy, their self-absorption alienates them from others when what they need most is human contact. Their selfishness, however, should not be interpreted as casual or as entirely voluntary: it is a matter of survival, for obsession with their own frail egos is the only means by which they may retain a semblance of sanity. Shannon's remark implies this, even while he acknowledges that seeing the problems of others may offer some emotional strength as well.

Many of Williams's plays feature at least one character at the point of emotional breakdown, and an inventory of these plays demonstrates the playwright's overwhelming interest in the mad and in society's view of madness. The playwright's first major success on Broadway, *The Glass Menagerie* (1945), offers a thinly veiled account of the author's own family life; it dramatizes Tennessee's "abandonment" of his sister Rose to madness and lobotomy.[17]

Although Laura's physical lameness provides the strongest visual indication of her social immobility, Laura's mental condition limits her as well, for after failing to complete high school, she withdraws from reality and lives in daydreams. Most critics assume that after Tom's departure, Laura will be institutionalized, thus living out the fate of her real-life counterpart, Rose. The play dramatizes the plight of the emotionally frail, but also conveys the extent to which those who love such people may bear the burden of guilt when the stronger ones escape from the trap of mental withdrawal. In Tom Wingfield, Williams creates a figure who has the strength to choose to live in the world, but suggests that this choice is not without its own kind of confinement. *The Glass Menagerie* in that sense provides the foundation for all that Williams will have to say about madness: the dangers of succumbing to emotional weakness, the tenuousness of escaping from that trap, and the oppressive nature of the confinement that haunts both those who submit and those who continue to struggle.

In a one-act play staged two years after *Menagerie,* Williams shows us the final moments before commitment. *Portrait of a Madonna* (1947) centers on Lucretia Collins, an aged unmarried woman who lives alone in a city apartment. This madonna is removed to an asylum after making public her hallucinations and her mental instability. She imagines that a married friend is making nighttime visits to her apartment and forcing himself sexually on her. She deludes herself that she is carrying his child. Since her pension has run out and the apartment manager is receiving complaints about the disturbances she causes, he regretfully decides to have her committed. Like Laura, Lucretia lives in a world of illusion, shutting herself off from society. Although her confinement in the apartment is voluntary, the strangeness of her complete withdrawal contributes to the decision those around her make to forcibly commit her.

A similar fate awaits the more compelling Blanche DuBois, the protagonist of *A Streetcar Named Desire* (1947). Having lost the family home and her job, Blanche comes to live with her sister and brother-in-law in a small apartment in New Orleans. When Blanche is raped by her brother-in-law, Stanley, and suffers a breakdown, her relatives send her to the state mental institution. Blanche suffers from illusions, like the other characters I have mentioned; her emotional instability is obvious from the opening scenes, but she fights to maintain control over herself, and is much more clear-sighted about her precarious position than Laura or Lucretia. She comments on her marginal status in the family, calling herself "one of those poor relations you've heard about," and she predicts her impending destruction when she claims that Stanley will destroy her: "The first time I laid eyes on him I thought to myself, that man is my executioner!" (I, 337, 351).[18]

In *Summer and Smoke,* entitled in an alternate version *Eccentricities of a Nightingale,* Alma Winemiller suffers from a nervous disorder; her mother, as Williams describes her in the early version of the play, "was a spoiled and selfish girl who evaded the responsibilities of later life by slipping into a state of perverse childishness."[19] In *Eccentricities,* Williams suggests that Alma's emotional condition is hereditary when Alma berates John Buchanan for rejecting her for someone more stable, with a better "family background, no lunacy in it, no skeletons in the closet . . . nothing peculiar, nothing eccentric! No—deviations!" (II, 80). Alma's name is Spanish for soul, and her inner conflict concerns the struggle she experiences between things of the body and things of the spirit. Part of her nervousness seems to stem from her inability to reconcile her dual nature. John Buchanan calls it her *doppelgänger* that affects her "nervous organization." Alma says her mother had a breakdown when Alma was still in high school, so that Alma's own nervous behavior partially results from enduring her mother's retreat into childhood. Williams describes her as "prematurely spinsterish" and prone to "nervous attacks."

After an excursion into other themes and other genres, Williams returns to the treatment of madness in his 1959 play *Suddenly Last Summer.* Catharine Holly, a young woman from New Orleans, is confined to a mental hospital because she has related a gruesome tale of her cousin, Sebastian's murder. Her aunt, Violet, the dead man's mother, entreats a psychiatrist from the state institution to perform an experimental procedure on her niece in order to silence her: lobotomy. *Suddenly,* more so than the earlier plays, does not assume Catharine's madness, but sets up a struggle between Violet and Catharine over their conflicting versions of Sebastian's life. This struggle involves the audience in deciding who is sane and who insane, thus emphasizing that these decisions are sometimes arbitrary. The play resembles *Streetcar* in its dramatization of the way that accusations of madness can tip the balance of power in a contest of wills between two characters, a theme to which Williams returns in *The Two-Character Play.*

In *The Night of the Iguana* (1961), Williams's characters populate a beach resort, a setting seemingly removed from all sources of mental tension, yet this drama explores a man's battle against madness. *Iguana* charts the nervous collapse of a Reverend Shannon, and is one of Williams's few full-length plays that focuses on a man's nervous condition. Williams includes a female character, Hannah Jelkes, who has experienced a near mental breakdown; she therefore possesses the empathy necessary to help Shannon wrestle with his "blue devils." The hotel is also the vacation spot for a group of German tourists; their rejoicing over successful German air strikes in Britain suggests the world's madness, Williams's most specific reference to world events in the plays discussed.

Felice in *The Two-Character Play* (1967) stands as another exception to the mainly female corpus of mad characters; he has been confined in the mental institution State Haven, as has his father before him. His mother used threats of institutionalization in efforts to control her husband, efforts that finally failed when the father killed his wife and himself. Throughout the play, brother and sister Felice and Clare argue about each other's insanity; they use one another's mental state in attempts to dominate the relationship. That both Shannon and Felice have the comfort of a female who shares their tendencies toward instability suggests that a madwoman can exist alone in a play, but that the madman must have a female cohort.[20]

In *Iguana,* although Shannon breaks down at a rustic hotel in Mexico, Maxine threatens to send him to the "Casa de Locos." He has been a resident there in the past, so in this he joins other Williams characters who have a history of mental illness: as Williams says of him, he is a "young man who's cracked up before, and is going to crack up again, perhaps repeatedly" (IV, 256). In a passage that does not appear in the final version, Shannon goes into some detail about his previous breakdowns, telling Hannah that he cracked up "two and a half times before," and that one time he was hauled off "to a Mexican bin for loonies the like of which I wouldn't regale you with a description of, Miss Jelkes honey."[21] He mentions his precarious mental condition throughout the play, explaining to Maxine and to Miss Fellowes that he is "at the end of his rope." Like Williams's women, Shannon is unable to control his sexual appetite, and Maxine's first words to him comment on the busload of females he is with, wondering, "How many you laid so far? Hah!" (IV, 255). When he relates the story of his defrocking to Hannah, he claims the young woman who came to see him to express her feelings for him had the "natural, or unnatural, attraction of one—lunatic for—another" (IV, 303).

Maxine immediately senses his instability, as noted in the following exchange in the typescript version:

Mrs. Faulk: How long have you been off it?
Shannon: I am not off the wagon.
Mrs. Faulk: I didn't mean the wagon, I meant your rocker.[22]

The published version deletes this remark, but has Maxine tell Shannon: "You're going to pieces, are you," to which Shannon replies, "No! Gone! Gone!" Maxine also asserts: "Shannon . . . you're not in a nervous condition to cope with this party" (IV, 259). Hannah appears peculiar to Maxine, who says of Hannah and her grandfather when they first appear together on the veranda: "They look like a pair of loonies" (IV, 278). In the typescript version, she adds to this by commenting, "This place gets them: every living eccentric"; she calls her hotel "a paradise for eccentrics" and a "mental hospital."[23] An isolated hotel in Mexico attracts those who seek a haven from the world, either emotional or financial; Shannon's appearance at the Costa Verde parallels the asylum that Blanche seeks with Stella and Stanley. Here the threat of commitment lingers, too, for Maxine threatens Shannon with a trip to "Casa de Locos." Her threat does not materialize; the play ends with Maxine attempting to convince Shannon to stay with her. The couple heads for the beach, with Maxine "half leading half supporting him" (IV, 374).

Six years after *Iguana*, Williams once again treated insanity as a central issue. *The Two-Character Play* unfolds in a theater where a brother and sister acting team have been abandoned by their company, who proclaim in a telegram that the pair are insane. Faced with an audience, they have no choice but to perform a play also called "The Two-Character Play," written by Felice with two characters, also named Felice and Clare. The inner play appears to be a biographical account of the couple's family life; their past is littered with family insanity, and their memories center around the murder/suicide of their parents. Felice has been institutionalized in the past, and both fear it as a distinct possibility for themselves in the future. When they are unable to escape the locked theater, but are equally incapable of a double suicide, they resolve to face the future one moment at a time by losing themselves in their play. *The Two-Character Play* differs from the earlier plays about madness in that the protagonists do not suffer from any serious threats of confinement in an institution, although they are accused of insanity by representatives of the outside world. This variation implies that these characters have found a retreat from the world that threatens them; as in *Iguana,* the end of the play suggests that the characters continue in whatever way they can. Felice and Clare's confinement in the theater suggests the limits of their freedom: they are safe here, however, from the judgment of others.

Other Williams plays of this period touch on madness and confinement, but in doing so either prove little more than repetitions of the earlier works, or do not coherently present mad characters worthy of sustained examination. *In the Bar of a Tokyo Hotel* (1969) and *The Red*

Devil Battery Sign (1976) feature Williams's characteristic nervous protagonists, but neither play contributes significantly to his career-long preoccupation with insanity. Only in one of his last full-length plays does Williams once more stake out the territory of the mad, this time by setting the stage in the very asylum that so many previous characters have feared. *Clothes for a Summer Hotel* (1980) is set in the mental asylum where Zelda Fitzgerald died in a fire in 1947. Relying on Nancy Mitford's biography of Zelda, the play explores the biographer's assertion that Scott discouraged Zelda's writing ambitions, a suppression that contributed to the latter's insanity. The action of the play revolves around a visit by Scott to Zelda; it interweaves past and present in their attempt to comprehend their failed marriage, Scott's struggles as a writer, and Zelda's institutionalization.

Throughout the plays here mentioned, the theme of confinement is inextricably interwoven with the theme of madness. From *The Glass Menagerie* to *Clothes for a Summer Hotel,* Williams's plays demonstrate his preoccupation with images of entrapment, and he uses the theater space to convey the constricting nature of the characters' worlds. He is not the first American dramatist to use the physical boundaries of the stage to convey the psychological constriction of the characters. Before Williams, Eugene O'Neill conceived sets that informed audiences about the characters' trapped lives.[24]

Confinement as a dominant image has retained its significance in contemporary theater, and is the subject of a book by Carol Rosen. Rosen examines plays set in a variety of confining institutions, including the hospital, the asylum, the prison, and the barracks.[25] The dramas she chooses "are madhouse plays which take us beyond curiosity, beyond voyeurism, to a poetic vision of an insane society akin to our own" (85). Although her asylum plays are not American, it is conceivable that a play such as *Streetcar,* with a most memorable mad protagonist, may have influenced the playwrights she studies. Despite Williams's frequent attention to confinement in his plays, Rosen refers only to *Small Craft Warnings,* categorizing that play as one of a group which dramatize a "state of impasse located in bars or restaurants, along with such works as O'Neill's *The Iceman Cometh*" (262).

Although O'Neill presented the limitations of modern life by his constricting sets, and introduced insanity to modern American drama in such plays as *Strange Interlude,* Williams was the first American playwright to inextricably link confinement and madness. From the 1940s to the end of his career, Williams portrayed insanity as the inevitable fate of a majority of his most memorable characters; they faced confinement as the result of their inability to retain their sanity. As Foucault writes of the period of the Great Confinement, from the middle of the seventeenth century to the end of the eighteenth, the "'insane' had as such a particular place in the world of confinement," their confinement "explained, or at least justified, by the desire to avoid scandal" (*M&C* 66). His study pertains to all forms of unreason, and the confinement of all these forms, but he claims:

In the general sensibility to unreason, there appeared to be a special modulation which concerned madness proper, and was addressed to those called, without exact semantic distinction, insane, alienated, deranged, demented, extravagant. (*M&C* 66)

Although written about a time hundreds of years before Williams's dramas, this depiction of the attitude towards the insane could be describing the characters of his plays. Not only are his mad characters defined with the same semantic looseness, both in the stage directions and in the dialogue, but the desire to avoid scandal by confining the source of the disturbance figures decisively in the outcomes of many of these plays. The situations of *Madonna, Streetcar, Suddenly,* and *Clothes* all depend on the impulse by some characters to contain the madness of another. When Foucault continues to say that confinement depends on recognizing "aspects of evil that have such a power of contagion, such a force of scandal that any publicity multiplies them infinitely," he might be describing the impulse that forces Violet Venable to silence her niece with a lobotomy, or that forces Stella to agree that Blanche be sent away.

Ironically, the shame and attempts at suppression of the madness that operate within the plays are counterbalanced by the public nature of the performance, for the mad person's ravings and eventual confinement become the public spectacle, with the theater audience as witness. This parallels a paradox that Foucault describes: in the Age of Reason, when unreason was silenced and confined, madness "became pure spectacle" in the displays of the mad that were popular in England and France (*M&C* 69). Williams's plays work as spectacle, for within the confined space of the theater, the play presents to the public characters whose behavior makes them unfit for societal interaction. We are able to view those who must be confined out of sight in the mental institution.

Williams's preoccupation with confinement is visible from his earliest plays. "Stairs to the Roof," written before 1941 and unpublished, contains an inscription following the title: "A Prayer for the Wild of Heart that are kept in Cages."[26] The play heavy-handedly provides a lesson to the middle class to cast off oppression and find the "stairs to the roof"; the author apologetically notes the abundance of didactic material in the play. A review of the 1947 world premiere, performed at the Pasadena Playhouse some six years after it was written, says that Williams "early in his writing career, had ideals" and "let off some of his steam in a message-type play."[27] In an author's note for the production, the playwright acknowledges that the play demonstrates "a moral earnestness which I cannot boast of today, and I think that moral earnestness is a good thing for any times but particularly for these times."[28] Despite its obvious flaws, the play provides evidence of Williams's sympathies for those "kept in cages." As he develops his interest in this theme, these "wild hearts" will increasingly become the emotionally disturbed; although "Stairs to the Roof" does not deal with mental illness, a number of aspects of this early effort are pertinent to my topic.

The opening stage directions describe a mechanized office scene, reminiscent of Elmer Rice's *The Adding Machine*. The workers make "rigid, machine-like motions above their imaginary desks," and the "girl at the filing cabinet (invisible) has the faraway stare of a schizophrenic as her arms work mechanically above the indexed cases" ("Stairs to the Roof" 5). The protagonist of the play prefigures some of Williams later nervous types, for Ben Murphy has the "nervous, defensive agility of a squirrel. Ten years of regimentation have made him frantic" (6). He tells his boss, Mr. Gum, that he has discovered the stairs to the roof because "I was stifling in here" (8). His employer informs him that your "work in this office has placed too many restrictions on your freedom" (9). Ben Murphy stands out among his fellow workers, and even his friends notice his peculiar nature: his friend Jim says, "Ben, you're off your nut!"; Jim tells his wife that Ben is "going to pieces," to which she replies: "Ben has always been an absolute screwball" (25). Late in the play, when Ben's wife leaves him, she tells her mother that Ben has "lost his mind and he's lost his job" (80). Ben's search for freedom and a chance for individual achievement sets him apart from the rest of his community and causes them to judge him as different. Within the context of the play, these comments pertain more to Ben's inability to live a regimented life than to mental imbalance, but they contain the seeds of Williams's later dramas, in which a character's desires lead to full-scale madness. "Stairs to the Roof" thus provides early evidence of the characteristics of confinement that lead in later plays to the protagonist's insanity. Seeking satisfaction beyond an approved system of behavior, in this case represented by an oppressive factory environment, leads to ostracism.

The play ends with a scene of the fabled roof that Ben discovered, with Ben and his female companion spirited away to a new star, to start a new and better civilization; this inspiring event leads the other workers of Continental Shirtmakers to rebel against the constricting rules of their employers. In the interim, Ben has inspired others, including his best friend, to escape from an unhappy life, and has freed the foxes from the zoo to resume their lives in the wild. The rather romantic conclusion offers an optimistic view of the ability to free oneself from confining situations, but optimism eludes Williams in the plays to come. The best of them omit the didacticism that flaws this early work, for they focus on the unhappiness and weakness of the individual. "Stairs to the Roof," however, reveals the building blocks of the later plays, indicating the playwright's interest in social injustice.

Many of Williams's plays take place in confined space, and the setting often suggests that the characters will face permanent confinement at the play's end. *The Glass Menagerie* is set in "one of those hive-like conglomerations of cellular living-units . . . symptomatic of the impulse of this largest and fundamentally enslaved section of American society to avoid fluidity and differentiation" (I, 143). Confinement figures as a major theme in this drama; Tom speaks frequently about the confinement that keeps him from fulfilling his dreams. In scene three, he berates his mother for the lack of privacy he feels in the apartment, telling her: "I've got no thing, no single thing—in my life that I can call my own!" (I, 161). He feels confined in his job, sarcastically wondering if Amanda thinks he wants to spend "fifty-five *years* down there in that—*celotex interior*! with—*fluorescent—tubes!*" (I, 163). When he returns from a night out, he brags to Laura about the magician who performed the coffin trick: "We nailed him into a coffin and he got out of the coffin without removing one nail" (I, 167). This, he claims, constitutes a "trick that would come in handy for me—get me out of this 2x4 situation!" (I, 167). Tom escapes from the oppressive apartment and the dead-end job, but does not find the freedom he expects, for he cannot forget his sister or the ties he feels to her, which bind him even in her absence.

Laura is voluntarily confined in the apartment, which, according to her mother, will lead to permanent confinement if she does not pursue a career or marriage. She will end up one of those "barely tolerated spinsters . . . stuck away in some little mouse-trap of a room" (I, 156). To the audience Laura's plight seems as constricted as the future her mother predicts, but if Laura's life proceeds as Lucretia's and Blanche's do, the "mouse-trap of a room" might well be in the state asylum. As Tom realizes, Laura is not just crippled: "In the eyes of others—strangers—she's terribly shy and lives in a world of her own and those things make her seem a little peculiar to people outside the house" (I, 187-88). Amanda's comment highlights Laura's social shortcomings, while Tom's remark focuses on her psychological ones: both assessments emphasize Laura's isolation.

Similar to *Menagerie* in its theme of confinement and isolation, *Portrait of a Madonna* is set in the sitting room of the apartment where Lucretia has lived for years, leaving only for errands and church activities. She has enforced her isolation by refusing to let others in; she lives a hermit's life, surrounded by old phonographs and newspapers. At the end of the play, she takes one last trip by way of the elevator (an enclosed space), to the locked ward of the asylum.

Although the set for *A Streetcar Named Desire* is somewhat more expansive, with both an interior and exterior playing space, the Kowalski apartment consists of only two rooms and a bath. Showing Blanche inside at the opening of the play, Eunice contrasts the small apartment to the "home-place" Blanche has come from, a "great big place with white columns" (I, 249). Blanche reacts to the apartment's size when Stella explains that it is too small to require a maid, "What? *Two* rooms, did you say?" (I, 255). Stella tells Stanley in scene two: "She wasn't expecting to find us in such a small place" (I, 271). Blanche sleeps in the kitchen/living room, with no door between it and the other room. She comments on the situation to Stella, worried about the decency of it, but what she does not mention is the lack of privacy. Her only opportunity for privacy is when she is locked in the bathroom, an even smaller enclosed space.

Blanche's move to the apartment is the latest in a series of relocations, each one to a smaller and less private space. We learn from the exposition that after she lost Belle Reve, she moved to the Flamingo Hotel; she calls it the "Tarantula Arms," a place where, she confesses to Mitch, "I brought my victims" (I, 386). Here Blanche is the captor, bringing men to her constricting web of desire, but her need to snare sexual companions leads to her own capture and ruin. The hotel room offers little privacy, for her behavior attracts the attention of the management, who evict her. Nonetheless, before she arrives in New Orleans, she still has a place of her own. In Elysian Fields this opportunity for solitude is gone. Blanche feels this lack keenly, speaking in scene ten of what she wishes for on her imagined trip with Shep Huntleigh: "When I think of how divine it is going to be to have such a thing as privacy once more—I could weep with joy!" (I, 396). Removed to the institution at the conclusion of the play, however, any chance of solitude evaporates. Her arrival at the Kowalski apartment, with a protest that "there's no door between the two rooms" foreshadows her final loss of privacy. The tiny and crowded Kowalski apartment is both way station and preparation for this final, confined space.

In *Asylums,* when explaining the kinds of forced interpersonal contact that occurs in "total institutions," Erving Goffman asserts:

The model for interpersonal contamination in our society is presumably rape; although sexual molestation certainly occurs in total institutions, there are many other less dramatic examples. Upon admission, one's on-person possessions are pawed and fingered by an official as he itemizes and prepares them for storage. (28)[29]

Blanche's stay with the Kowalskis foreshadows the more violating aspects of institution life. In scene two, the day after Blanche's arrival, Stanley "paws and fingers" the contents of Blanche's trunk, with as little sensitivity as an asylum guard. Blanche protests against his appropriation of her love-letters, a most intimate possession, for she cries: "The touch of your hands insults them!" and "Now that you've touched them I'll burn them!" (I, 282). The last remark implies that she can no longer protect her personal property, but prefers to destroy it rather than have it contaminated by others. Stanley's rifling through her belongings foreshadows what the officials at the institution might do, in admission procedures that "can be seen as the institution's way of getting him [the patient or recruit] ready to start living by house rules" (Goffman 49). The parallel Goffman draws between such institutional practices and rape, moreover, suggests the connection of this violation by Stanley to the ultimate violation he commits in scene ten. By raping Blanche, he not only brings on her commitment, he prepares her for any and all personal contamination she may face in the asylum.

Another aspect of the institutions that Goffman discusses has some relevance to Blanche's situation, for he speaks of the "barrier that total institutions place between the inmate and the wider world" (14). In total institutions, communication with the outside world is either forbidden or strictly controlled; if allowed, such freedoms as telephone privileges or letter exchanges are strictly monitored. Blanche makes two abortive attempts to use the telephone, both times to reach Shep Huntleigh, who she imagines will rescue her. The first time occurs in scene five, when she attempts to arrange an escape for herself and Stella, in the aftermath of the poker night and Stanley's violence. She fails to operate the phone successfully, while Stella languidly looks on, providing simple instructions for dialing which Blanche cannot master: "I can't dial, I'm too—" (I, 317). She reconsiders her approach, deciding to write the telegram down before phoning it in, but once more finds her tactics inadequate, for she "smashes the pencil on the table and springs up" (I, 318).

Immediately before the rape in scene ten, Blanche tries unsuccessfully to use the phone to contact her imagined savior, but only manages to hoarsely whisper a vague cry for help: "Caught in a trap. Caught in— Oh!" (I, 400). Stanley's emergence from the bathroom causes Blanche to break off her plea, and the line goes dead. The scene suggests that of an inmate defying the authorities in order to seek outside assistance, and being caught in the act of transgression. Blanche is as isolated from the world here, in her relatives' apartment, as she soon will be in the institution.

Another constricting environment suggests confinement in *Suddenly Last Summer*. The play takes place in the jungle-like garden of the Venable home. The setting recalls the quotation from the Song of Solomon that Williams uses for the epigraph to *The Two-Character Play:* "A garden enclosed is my sister . . . a spring shut up, a fountain sealed." The film version of *Suddenly* (screenplay by Gore Vidal) moves some of the action to the private asylum where Catharine Holly has been confined; contrasting the two versions highlights the stage version's success in conveying an atmosphere of confinement, for the film seems more mobile, although it contains scenes in the institution, the ultimate location of confinement.

Williams also uses aspects of the total institution to convey Catharine's predicament, the most obvious being the references to various forms of treatment: drug therapy, insulin shock treatments, electric shock treatments, and lobotomy. When Catharine appears at the opening of scene two, with the nun who accompanies her from St. Mary's, her first action onstage has her taking a cigarette from a box on the table and lighting it. Goffman lists smoking as one of the "minor activities that one can execute on one's own on the outside," which becomes, in the institution, an act requiring permission from the staff (41). As Goffman argues: "This obligation not only puts the individual in a submissive or suppliant role 'unnatural' for an adult but also opens up his line of action to interceptions by staff" (41). The sister repeatedly demands that Catharine put out the cigarette, ignoring pleas from Catharine that their removal from hospital grounds might allow for a relaxation of hospital policy. Catharine makes no headway with this line of argument, however, and shows her frustration by extinguishing the cigarette in the nun's outstretched hand. This establishes Catharine's character as willful, while highlighting the personal restrictions of asylum life. Even when away from the hospital, the patient's most ordinary privileges are limited by the restrictions of the total institution. Catharine's behavior is more understandable in light of the claim that Goffman makes: "Many of these potential gratifications are carved out of the flow of support that the inmate had previously taken for granted" (49). Such common acts as smoking a cigarette take on heightened significance, "re-establishing relationships with the whole lost world and assuaging withdrawal symptoms from it and one's lost self" (Goffman 49). Thus, Catharine's first act in the play signals her desire to take control of her environment and assert herself as an autonomous member of society. The nun's refusal to allow this freedom, and the doctor's subsequent granting permission to smoke, signifies their different perspectives on Catharine's role.

The Night of the Iguana continues the theme of constriction, even though the action unfolds on the veranda of a Mexican hotel, overlooking the sea. In the directions for the set, Williams specifies that the veranda should be enclosed by a railing (or that at least this should be suggested), and that the bedrooms be narrow cubicles opening onto the veranda (IV, 253). However, Williams also suggests that the "style of the setting should be free and lyric"; the combination of the confinement of the veranda and the freedom of the set, with the ocean just beyond, suggests that this play might present the possibility of escape. The set also includes "a path down to the beach," the path that Maxine and Shannon take at the end of the play, with the promise of freedom that they might find together (IV, 253). However, before Shannon can achieve his freedom, he spends the night tied in a hammock, his straitjacket, while Hannah cures him with conversation and poppy-seed tea, a treatment of "psychotherapy" and "drugs."

Both Shannon and Hannah have struggled with "blue devils" or "spooks": they have kept a step ahead of these tormentors by running around the world. Shannon's bag is a "beat-up Gladstone covered with travel stickers from all over the world" (IV, 256). Hannah and Nonno have "ancient luggage fantastically plastered with hotel and travel stickers indicating a vast range of wandering" (IV, 286). In one of the earlier versions, Shannon tells Maxine that he "can't stay still and can't afford to travel without conducting these tours!"[30] When Maxine has Shannon tied in the hammock, he implores Hannah to untie him, for he "can't stand being tied up . . . It makes me panicky" (IV, 343). In the earlier version of the play, he lies in the hammock, but is not tied in it; this addition provides the concrete stage image of Shannon's confinement.

Hannah and Shannon furnish the most striking evidence of how Williams's creations seek to avoid confinement by moving around, but there are other examples. Sebastian Venable seeks freedom in travel, and takes an extensive trip every summer in order to write his one poem a year. Although Blanche does not travel the world, and her journey is as much a spiral downward as it is an escape, her trunk is a central image in her play. Its constant presence onstage indicates that her life has become transitory, that she cannot permanently reside in the Kowalski home.

Felice and Clare in *The Two-Character Play* have traveled on tour for a long time; their life of travel has become no more than a blur to Clare, who claims they were on their way there "interminably," and that she does not have "any idea or suspicion of where we are now except we seem to be somewhere like nowhere."[31] Felice indicates how long and far they have traveled when he asks Clare if she wants "to cross back over forty, fifty frontiers on wooden benches in third class coaches?"[32] Like Hannah and Nonno, Felice and Clare are artists who make a living on the road, who find their talents less than appreciated at this point in their lives, and who have come to the "end of their rope." The theater that they occupy at present may be, for them, the place for stopping. At the end of *Iguana,* Hannah speaks of this need to quit wandering: "Oh, God, can't we stop now?" (IV, 375).

Clothes for a Summer Hotel picks up on some themes explored in *The Two-Character Play:* the inextricable bonds of the protagonist couple (in this case married, not brother and sister), the characters' awareness of the theatrical situation, the limited playing space (here an asylum, although the action shifts in time through memory). Called a "ghost play" by Williams (the characters are dead), Scott and Zelda look with some detachment on their lives. If the setting does indicate their afterlife, the institution where Zelda died has become the couple's final destination, suggesting the central image of confinement in both lives. That the action unfolding is a drama is noted immediately by Gerald Murphy, who tells Scott: "It will all be over in—one hour and forty-five minutes," the real time of the play (*Clothes* 3). Zelda's first meeting with Scott also draws on the theatrical nature of the event, for she asks the Intern, "How shall I play it?" (7). The players are locked into the events of the performance, and Zelda's attempts to avoid a confrontation with Scott are futile; she is surprised by this obligation, for she "thought that obligations stopped with death!" (8). Throughout the play, Zelda comments on the confinement of the asylum, calling it a "cage," announcing "feeding time at the zoo"; she speaks of the "barred door," and of being "caught and led into and locked!" Her final words denote her separation from Scott, which is accomplished by the institution setting: "The gates are iron, they won't admit you or ever release me again" (77). Like the other plays of this study, *Clothes* concerns itself with characters who are trapped by their present circumstances into a course of action that tests their courage. In this work, the characters are limited by the rules of the asylum, and by the choices of their past.

The plays under examination all focus to some degree on the dangers that a harsh world presents to its most vulnerable inhabitants; no clear escape exists, for the characters are equally threatened by the confinement which signifies the removal from a society in which they cannot function. If the world offers no protection for these characters, one wonders what kind of world it is; does Williams use these characters, their search for freedom as well as their ultimate confinement, to comment on a world that contains no solace? Allan Ingram asserts in his discussion of madness and language in the eighteenth century, that "the opposition between the professionals in the debate about madness comes down to the difference between two attitudes: suppression, and endorsement" (17). His distinction between these two attitudes is descriptive of outlooks on madness pertinent to Williams's plays.

Those of suppressive tendencies looked upon madness as a departure from the norm of a healthy mind, though they might well differ as to what in the mind was responsible for that departure—impaired judgement, for example, or a diseased imagination. Those more inclined to endorsement saw in the particular form of madness a response to a set of circumstances, a way of life, or a social system. (*Ingram 18*)

Perhaps interpretation of Williams's mad characters may combine these views, but it might be useful to give one view precedence, to illuminate the thrust of the playwright's argument about the world, and his characters' ability to explain the world to the audience. For, as Ingram maintains, at "bottom, suppression and endorsement differed over whether the experience of madness contained any kind of truth" (18). The implications are thus: "If madness was saying something about normal life, and was also a commentary upon itself, then the mad could offer important clues for the understanding both of themselves and of the world of the sane" (18).

The question that follows from this supposition, in Williams's drama, is: what clues does he provide about the world that has rejected and confined these characters we are preparing to study? Is the sensitive and insecure individual driven to madness because of the shortcomings of the society? Brooks Atkinson called *Suddenly Last Summer* Williams's "most devastating statement about corruption in the world, and his most decisive denial of the values by which most people try to live."[33] Writing about *Streetcar,* Harold Clurman writes that Williams is a "poet of frustration, and what his play says is that aspiration, sensitivity, departure from the norm are battered, bruised, and disgraced in our world today," and that the play "speaks of a poet's reaction to life in our country."[34]

The world in Williams's plays is usually represented by a few characters, who are unlike the sensitive protagonists. In *The Glass Menagerie,* Jim is the "emissary from the world," touched but perplexed by Laura's insular life, enthusiastically but foolishly encouraging her to overcome her "inferiority complex" and bolster her self-esteem. He also tries to sell Tom "a bill of goods" in the form of a public speaking class. Although Jim's own career dreams have not yet and may never materialize, nonetheless he is the only character in the play whose ties to the world are secure. That he should represent society, as lacking as he is in success, does not speak well for the world of the play. After stimulating Laura's desire for love, then abruptly breaking her heart, Jim leaves the Wingfield home unaware of the disappointment and tragedy his visit has precipitated. Unlike other representatives of the world in Williams's plays, Jim inflicts pain unintentionally; he does, however, embody the insensitivity and smallness of the world that the more sensitive characters shrink from. For Laura, Jim symbolizes the pain and risk of opening her heart to others; after Jim departs, she quickly closes up once more. For Tom, Jim's life embodies the smallness of a high-school hero turned shipping clerk, whose adventurous days ended when the cast of *The Pirates of Penzance* gave their final performance. Jim's world is not the menacing world of some of the later plays, but it is inadequate in encouraging the shy or the sensitive. Williams's later plays more often present a world that threatens destruction for the overwrought protagonists who struggle to survive.

In his best plays, the world that surrounds and threatens the mad person is at once menacing and cruel, but attractive to the audience in its power and vitality. Such is the world of Elysian Fields, epitomized by Stanley Kowalski, the proud peacock who presides over his corner of the quarter. As sympathetic as we are to Blanche's rejection of Stanley's coarse, uneducated, and vulgar lifestyle, his world dominates; allegiance to him entails hanging "back with the brutes," but as Stella realizes, this constitutes survival. The spirit and liveliness of the French Quarter are compromised by domestic violence and street crime, and Blanche's mad ravings in scene ten are matched and perhaps outdone by the criminal actions on the street behind the scrim. If Stanley's world is the "sane" one, this sanity includes indiscriminate violence and brutality. We are left to choose between two forms of existence that have serious drawbacks, and our inability to embrace either leaves the reader or audience uncomfortably stranded, which may be Williams's intention.

Williams stated that the Nazis in *The Night of the Iguana* correspond to Stanley in *Streetcar*. As background figures, he says, "I feel that they offer a vivid counterpoint—as world conquerors—to the world-conquered protagonists of the play."[35] Faced with the similarity that Williams suggests, we see that, for the audience, the *Iguana* version of the "mortal combat between the Blanches and the Stanleys" is more heavily weighted in favor of the Blanches. The Nazis are little more than, as Shannon puts it, a "little animated cartoon by Hieronymus

Bosch," less attractive than the least attractive quality of the world Stanley represents. Although *Iguana* is set in 1940, so that the Germans in the play are rejoicing over the Nazi victories, the audience's knowledge of Nazi crimes against humanity prevent these characters from incurring favor. If these Germans are the emissaries of the world, then the world in this play has indeed gone mad. Only slightly less attractive is the character Judith Fellowes, the leader of the Baptist schoolteacher group that Shannon has been squiring around Mexico. Her nagging condemnation of Shannon, attacking him for everything from his deficiencies as tour guide to his "seduction" of Charlotte, makes it easy for us to empathize with his nervous condition.

The suggestion that Williams makes is that a person's natural reaction in these circumstances would be to break down in the face of this harsh, critical world. Society's brutal nature offers little opportunity for peaceful existence; those who lack the necessary survival techniques are destroyed or ostracized, or both.

2

Captive Maids: Women and Madness

Madness is the impasse confronting those whom cultural condition-
ing has deprived of the very means of protest or self-affirmation.
—Shoshana Felman
"Women and Madness: The Critical Phallacy"

Tennessee Williams is admired for his ability to create memorable
women characters in his plays; his critics in turn, have attempted to categorize and analyze these women in a vast variety of ways. Robert
Emmet Jones divided the playwright's early heroines into genteel relics
and healthy earth goddesses ("Heroines"). Signi Falk increases the categories by consigning mothers (of the Southern variety) into their own
group (169). Using Jungian varieties of the "Great Mother" figure,
Nancy Tischler rescinds their heroine status and labels them "A Gallery
of Witches" ("Gallery"). Focusing on their situations at the time of the
action of the play, Louise Blackwell analyzes them in terms of four categories of predicaments. While acknowledging Williams's ability to
create "an incredibly varied portrait gallery of female types," Durant da
Ponte nevertheless proceeds to group them. In an article that attempts a
psychoanalysis of Blanche, while admitting the impossibility of doing so
to a fictional character, Philip Weissman concludes that Blanche, Willie
from *This Property Is Condemned,* and Mrs. Hardwick-Moore of *The
Lady of Larkspur Lotion* are "derivatives of a single image in the
author's unconscious" (178).

Although these examples do not exhaust the range and quantity of
articles on women and Williams, they are representative of the discussions within the critical canon on this American playwright, particularly
on the first two decades of his work. Their insights notwithstanding,
these essays share a tendency to reduce Williams's characters to types, in
order to satisfy the particular pattern the critic wishes to construct. My
study demonstrates that the critics' emphasis on establishing likeness
often limits and impedes their explorations of character. Most of the
studies mentioned above focus on "reading Williams' plays as sexual
dramas in which the southern gentlewoman and the natural woman rep-

resent respectively the spirit and the flesh" (McGlinn 510). While attitudes towards sexuality are an essential component of character formation in these plays, emotional makeup is another crucial factor. By dwelling on sexual natures alone, those who have written about Williams's women have been directed by a discussion of these, rather than by issues of insanity. Most have acknowledged, however briefly, that insanity awaits these women almost as often as death awaits Shakespeare's tragic heroes.

A brief review of the articles I have mentioned provides the necessary background. Philip Weissman relies on the tactic that seems to be symptomatic of Williams's critics, a tactic that unfortunately results in undermining the range of the Williams's canon: he conflates the characters.

With only the minimal sacrifice of creative reality it is possible to see the thirteen year old Willie grown into the thirty year old Blanche du Bois whom we have last seen ejected from her last refuge and institutionalized, emerging in a final scene of deterioration and hopelessness ten years later and older as Mrs. Hardwick-Moore, whose Belle Reve plantation becomes a Brazilian rubber plantation, whose oil king becomes a rubber king and whose prostitutional promiscuity has become a dismal reality. (180)

Da Ponte, on the other hand, conflates Alma with Blanche, for "Alma, in effect, is Blanche DuBois at the beginning of the downhill slide to degradation. Blanche is Alma at the end of the road" (19). He makes this claim while simultaneously defending Williams as a master of ambiguity, a playwright who creates characters that leave the audience guessing about what will happen to them. The contradiction arises, perhaps, out of da Ponte's insistence on proving the stereotype, rather than allowing for the differences that make comparing the women a complex and fruitful endeavor. Da Ponte also claims that the characters Williams created "would seem to be projections of his own distorted personality, frightened, timid, groping, highly sensitive, somewhat neurotic dreamers who, like their creator, are unable to adjust to the harsh realities of a world of crass materialism and brute strength" (13).

One of the most naive assertions that a literary critic can make is to insist that the characters are really just some aspect of the author. This approach limits critical inquiry about the works; in this case, if the plays tell us only about Williams himself, then they hold interest only for those who wish to know more about the playwright (and there are volumes about the man himself, as well as collected letters, and, of course, his infamous memoirs). Although biographical interpretation is but one of a variety of approaches, it has too often dominated the critical methods applied to Williams; this has resulted in a restriction of insight, rather than the expansion we rightly expect from literary interpretation. I argue that the plays compel and interest audiences and readers because they are about *other* people, they are about men and women and their emotional lives, and they present possibilities for exploration that do not hinge on divulging information about the personality of the author.

In "Tennessee Williams and the Predicament of Women," Louise Blackwell admits that Williams has created a variety of women characters, or, more accurately, that "Williams is careful to distinguish the underlying reasons for their behavior" (101). All the women are frustrated in their search for a satisfying sexual relationship, and perhaps this similarity invites critics to compare them, but Blackwell does insist that analysis of the plays "reveals subtle differences in the cause of their frustration, so that there is not as much similarity among the characters as is often supposed" (101). Her subsequent discussion includes grouping the women into a number of types, while allowing more for variations than do da Ponte or Weissman, but she finally asserts that the the major female characters (in plays written through *The Night of the Iguana*) pursue an identical goal: a mate, and therefore the assurance of "satisfactory sexual adjustment" (106).[1]

Nancy Tischler, with her "Gallery of Witches," uses Jungian archetypes of the Feminine. Applying a version outlined in *The Great Mother* by Erich Neumann, Tischler categorizes Williams's female characters according to four poles of development: the good Mother, the terrible Mother, the positive transformative character and the negative transformative character ("Gallery" 495). Although Tischler groups Williams's women, she manages not to compress them in order to strengthen her arguments. Her essay begins, however, with a notation on the often-quoted categories of Signi Falk's discussion of the females in the plays: southern gentlewomen, southern wenches, and southern mothers. Her efforts to reconsider and expand these groupings are, nevertheless, defined in part by Falk's definitions. Falk's own attempts at expansion of the influential Robert Emmet Jones essay on the early heroines retains intact Jones's thesis of the southern woman; this basic premise, therefore, remains constant throughout most of the criticism written about Williams's women characters.

Jones seems to be most influential in establishing the trends of grouping the women into categories and associating them with the South; his essay relies heavily on the myth of the Old South as set forth in W. J. Cash (211).[2] No doubt Jones, in proposing that Williams's early heroines are relics of the antebellum southern aristocrat, makes some salient points about Williams's art that have been confirmed and often expanded over the years. Certainly, many of Williams's heroines can be viewed in their southern context, "a world of yesterday and today, practically never of tomorrow. The characters of Williams always look to the past for their salvation" (Jones 212).

However, like the other critics I have mentioned, who analyze the characters by conflating them, this overriding presentation of the South leads Jones to remark that the neurotic southern white woman is the same character in a number of plays. Allowing for the differences in their ages, he claims that the four women he is discussing, "Alma, Cassandra, Blanche, and Amanda—have much in common and in fact, are really the same person at different stages of life" (Jones 212). The critic then follows through with this compression of the four women by discussing one of them: Blanche, very obviously the best choice for an examination of the cavalier Old South, since she is fresh off the plantation, and speaks of it often.

Although Blanche's southern identity is important to her play, and Jones makes some important points about southern society in order to explain the sexual dilemma of these women, by concentrating on their southern qualities he undermines the power of these dramas to present convincing portraits of women that transcend the southern realm. My discussion seeks to break out of this pattern that conflates the characters into one and forces that omni-character to represent the South of a certain period, for I wish to present the women characters in Williams's plays as individuals, individuals who are women first and southern women second, rather than the other way around.

An examination of some of the texts written about women and madness will show that time period and place do not much alter the fate of women who display qualities that do not conform to the society they live in; in several periods and locales, one common way that members of our society attempt to control these women is by designating them mad. For theories of madness, I refer to a cross section of important studies of women and madness in various disciplines, reliant both on feminist study and on the recent philosophical and sociological interest in madness. The texts on this subject are strikingly similar in their proposition that madness is a political category, that the diagnosis and confinement of women for mental illness arises out of the need to control certain kinds of behavior not conducive to society's ends.

Most of the texts that treat the subject of women and madness acknowledge that various studies of modern patterns of institutionalization indicate that women more often than men suffer from mental illness. Although this parallels the fact that most of the characters in Williams's plays who go mad are female, I would not hold this assertion to be a certainty. My research indicates that most psychologists or sociologists who argue this point ultimately face the reality that there is no way to prove this statement; statistics gathered from institutions and community health centers can only record the people who seek help from professionals, not the ones who do not.

To discount these statistics as questionable, however, is not to deny that women and madness are often linked both in theoretical texts and in literature, including Williams's plays. Etymology provides evidence of the association in the word hysteria, which derives from *hustera,* "womb," for hysteria was once thought to be caused by uterine disturbances. Elaine Showalter speaks of the connection between "women" and "madness":

By far the more prevalent view, however, sees an equation between femininity and insanity that goes beyond statistical evidence or the social conditions of women. Contemporary feminist philosophers, literary critics, and social theorists have called attention to the existence of a fundamental alliance between "woman" and "madness." (3)

A brief survey of the literature on women and insanity indicates that despite the fact that these scholars study women in different cultures and in different time periods, some common remarks about women and insanity link them. All the texts focus on the relationship of society to the madwoman, and argue that in many cases what is called mental illness could be better defined as the demonstration of a troublemaker, a disruption of the social and cultural orders. Yannick Ripa notes that in nineteenth-century France, committing people to an institution was a way to control "dangerousness," to maintain order in Paris, for the "slightest threat to public order was seen as a danger which had to be contained" (15). Ripa distinguishes between the fate of men and women who exhibited aggressive public behavior, noting that being aggressive to the police "would lead men to prison and women to the asylum" (16). She also maintains that "women who refused to conform and genuine cases of madness could be mixed up, and rebellion could become a symptom of mental illness" (15).

Philip W. Martin, in his book *Madwomen in Romantic Writing,* cites the frequency with which women in literature are designated insane, explaining that this frequency may be the result of the definition of madness as the antithesis of reason, for madness "thus gives meaning to reason and finds itself easily allied to woman in the system of difference which grants self-justifying presence to a specifically patriarchal normality" (Martin 6). Martin goes on to justify his premise by quoting extensively from medical texts of the period, which refer to a mythology in which women are naturally predisposed to madness (28-48).

In *The Psychopathology of Women,* Ihsan Al-Issa, like Ripa, proposes that different attitudes about the appropriateness of aggression and sexual roles lead to different treatment and attitudes toward those who exhibit the aggressive behavior:

Sex stereotypes may affect the definition of mental illness in such a way that breaking away from one's sex role (sex-role reversal) may take on negative valuation and be considered abnormal—for example, aggression, overt sexuality, and intellectuality in women . . . women who expressed aggression were seen as more disturbed than men who did so. (Al-Issa 26-27)

Phyllis Chesler in her book *Women and Madness* states that for women, madness is sometimes "a doomed search for potency" and concludes, very similarly to Ripa and Al-Issa, that "the search often involves 'delusions' or displays of physical aggression, grandeur, sexuality, and emotionality. . . . Such traits in women are feared and punished in patriarchal mental asylums" (31).[3]

Ripa devotes a large portion of her text to a discussion of family structure. She argues that women who did not fulfill the expected roles of wife and mother were then in danger of being committed, for their refusal or inability to accept or fill these roles was interpreted as madness. Her discussion of spinsters is particularly relevant to most of the plays I have chosen by Williams, for his characters are frequently women who are unmarried or widowed and whose tenuous position in their families, without a husband to protect or support them, renders them more susceptible to the charge and penalty of mental illness.[4]

The pervasiveness of the attitudes about the connection between women and madness makes Williams's use of this mythology understandable. His plays utilize the stereotypes about women and madness that influence cultural attitudes toward women: his madwoman character embodies the hysterical, unstable figure whose behavior seems to justify her commitment. We might consider, however, whether he presents these stereotypes in order that we question them. Is the "punishment" justly administered in these dramas, or do those who seek to categorize these women as mad do so because of their own fears? What kind of society endorses suppression of those women who do not conform to the narrow confines of wife and mother, and masks that suppression as therapeutic and caring?

In the plays that I include in my study of women and madness, the women are unmarried, except for Zelda Fitzgerald in *Clothes for a*

Summer Hotel. In *The Glass Menagerie* Amanda warns Laura about the difficulty of an unmarried life of dependency:

what becomes of unmarried women who aren't prepared to occupy a position . . . barely tolerated spinsters living upon the grudging patronage of sister's husband or brother's wife! . . . little birdlike women without any nest—eating the crust of humility all their life! (I, 156)

In accounting for these women and their madness, therefore, I will consider not only the ways that we see their mental condition as fragile, or how they represent the portrait of the rebellious or "dangerous" woman, but to what extent their social and economic conditions place them in jeopardy. By reading the plays with an eye to the theories outlined here, we may better understand the madwomen characters Williams creates; also, we may assess to what extent the playwright protests the role as patient that society assigns them.

A *Streetcar Named Desire* best embodies the playwright's vision of the madwoman, for in no other play does Williams dramatize a woman's mental decline and fall so completely. Lucretia, in the one-act *Portrait of a Madonna,* faces the same fate as Blanche, but that play's action takes place on the day of her commitment; we hear commentary only from the hotel workers on how and why Lucretia faces institutionalization. In *Suddenly Last Summer,* the details of Catharine Holly's confinement are told in retrospect, and although Violet's anger threatens Catherine with a lobotomy, the latter's release from her confinement is suggested, if she has convinced the doctor that she tells the truth about Sebastian's death. Although both Hannah and Shannon talk about their "blue devils" or "spooks" in *The Night of the Iguana*, the action is restricted to the deck of Maxine's beach resort; Shannon is confined to the hammock during the play, but this is the closest any of the characters comes to confinement in the stage present. Moreover, Shannon's breakdown has occurred prior to the opening of the play, and so the audience does not witness the escalation into madness. The action of *Clothes for a Summer Hotel* unfolds in the asylum where Zelda Fitzgerald spent her final years; while the well-publicized lives of Zelda and Scott provide us with background events leading up to her institutionalization, and part of the play consists of flashback to an earlier time, the play does not dramatize precisely what causes Zelda's confinement.

A predecessor to *Streetcar, Madonna* was produced by Hume Cronyn in Los Angeles in early 1947; it deals with some of the same issues that Williams develops more fully in *Streetcar.*[5] Miss Lucretia Collins, a "middle-aged spinster," is removed from her home in a city apartment house and taken to the state institution by a doctor and nurse who closely resemble the ones who come for Blanche. A less complex play than *Streetcar,* dramatizing only the last moments of freedom for Lucretia and narrating the circumstances of her commitment, *Madonna* nevertheless provides important evidence for the theories of women and madness that I have introduced.

At the opening of the play, Lucretia has attracted the attention of the management of her apartment house by insisting that the manager, Mr. Abrams, call the police to arrest the intruder who has been coming into her apartment regularly and "indulging his senses" (VI, 109). The intruder is imaginary; Mr. Abrams recognizes this, for it is not the first time that Lucretia has made this allegation. She claims this intruder is a man from her past, the man she was in love with as a young girl; he became involved with and married someone else.

In the character of Lucretia, we have an example of the Crazy Jane or Crazy Kate figure that Elaine Showalter mentions in the introduction of *The Female Malady:* "a docile and harmless madwoman who devoted herself singlemindedly to commemorating her lost lover" (13). Crazy Jane was the most popular of Romantic madwomen, and frequently appeared in ballads, melodramas, and paintings during this period. Showalter goes on to explain that the Crazy Jane image even influenced drawings of asylum madwomen, and these plates show "standardized female portraits in the Crazy Jane style . . . they are shown in elaborate caps and bonnets, like the millinery models in the ladies' annals" (14).

Lucretia not only pines over a long-lost lover (although her narrative about the past hints that he was never a lover, never more than the object of a schoolgirl crush), but she also dresses in the Crazy Jane style: "Her hair is arranged in curls that would become a young girl and she wears a frilly negligee which might have come from a hope chest of a period considerably earlier" (VI, 109).

When the porter and the elevator boy arrive at her apartment door, their conversation informs the audience of Lucretia's present circumstances. She has been a recluse in the apartment for years, seldom leaving, never allowing anyone entry. The porter tells the younger man, who wonders if she has money stashed away, that a monthly pension supported Miss Collins for years and that the checks have recently stopped coming. Although she has caused commotions in the past, forbidding the repair people to enter her apartment, the manager will evict her only when she is destitute. Like Blanche, who became desperate and liable to expulsion from Laurel when she lost Belle Reve, Lucretia must face a future at the asylum when she can no longer pay the rent on an apartment that kept her safe from the world, and even, apparently, from complaining neighbors. She was not safe, however, from her overactive imagination.

Lucretia's economic condition is tied to her unmarried status; she has no husband or children to care for her; once her pension is gone, there is nothing to keep the manager from turning her out, and the asylum seems an appropriate place to send her. Twice in the play we become aware of how alone Lucretia is: the porter tells the elevator boy that she has lived alone since her mother died fifteen years previously; Lucretia, in calling for the police to protect her from her imaginary intruder, explains that she is not "fortunate enough to have a father and brothers who can take care of the matter privately without any scandal" (VI, 119).

Having no male relatives to shield her from scandal also means that she has no male relatives to save her from the asylum. In Lucretia's case, her unmarried status leaves her particularly vulnerable because she has never had a career or any income other than her pension. The porter quotes Lucretia to explain to the elevator boy that she has never concerned herself with her economic situation, for "Southern ladies was never brought up to manage finanshul affairs" (VI, 111). She told Mr. Abrams this when she turned over her monthly checks to him; by doing so, she places herself in his hands, and he takes the responsibility seriously. When the pension runs out, he takes it upon himself to seek a contribution from her church so that she can stay on at the apartment house, which temporarily delays her institutionalization.

When she causes a major disturbance, however, the manager decides to have her evicted. Since Lucretia gave herself to the care of Mr. Abrams, he is the one who calls for the doctor and nurse to take her away. When Lucretia gives up the right to handle her own affairs, by proclaiming that ladies were not raised to handle money matters, she gives up the right to decide what happens to her. Her limited grasp of reality makes her even more susceptible to her fate, for she is unaware, until the last few moments of the play, that she is to be taken from the apartment house.

Lucretia's psychosis also leads her to think herself pregnant by her intruder, who is the man she was in love with when she was a young girl, and whose rejection of her contributed to her flight from reality. From her narration of past events, we gather that she was enamored of a young man who was fond of her but preferred the company of another more outgoing girl. Lucretia describes the other girl as "shameless" and a "common little strumpet."

The young man married the other girl, and Lucretia never recovered from it, telling the porter and the elevator boy how difficult it was for her to go on living in the same community with the couple. She speaks of having to walk by their house after Sunday services at the church, how they watched her from the porch and talked about her, the woman remarking to her husband about the passing of the "poor old maid—that loves you!" (VI, 121). This remark points out that Lucretia is a lovelorn spinster, but it also implies that Lucretia's infatuation with the young man was never taken seriously by him or by anyone, except for Lucretia.

Once we know the history, Lucretia's delusions that he has come back after all these years, breaking into her apartment and forcing himself on her, become all the more pathetic. Like Blanche, Lucretia dwells on a past love experience that ended badly, but while Blanche's guilt about her homosexual husband's death does stem from her choosing unwisely in love, and from the cruel things that she said to him, at least she had a relationship with a man who cared for her. Lucretia's imagined beau, on the other hand, was never more than a friend to her, although Lucretia has convinced herself that the other girl lured him away with her sexuality.

Another distinction between Blanche and Lucretia is that while they both escape the loneliness of their situation by dwelling on sexual encounters, Blanche actually does meet men: "intimacies with strangers was all I seemed able to fill my empty heart with" (I, 386). Lucretia's sexual "encounters" with the man from her past are fictional, and she imagines the encounters are forced. Lucretia situates herself within her fantasies in such a way that she can remain morally above reproach, a reflection of her strict religious upbringing and her aversion to sexuality.

She is horrified by sexuality, and this repulsion seems to be a symptom of her emotional disturbance, for it controls her life to the extent that she cannot pursue a real relationship; her rape fantasy, however, indicates that she is preoccupied with sex. She also fantasizes that she is pregnant. Her confinement at the end of the play, therefore, alludes to confinement during pregnancy; this allusion is heightened by the illegitimate status of her "baby," for it suggests that she needs to go away to maintain secrecy about her condition.

Her delusions about pregnancy indicate that despite her contempt for the woman that her "lover" married, she seeks to align herself with the woman, who, as Lucretia has told the two men, had six children with Richard. Even though she denigrates the wife's character throughout the play, she speaks of her "in white, so fresh and easy, her stomach round with a baby, the first of the six" (VI, 122). Lucretia describes the woman in motherhood as pure and lovely, despite the other disparaging remarks she makes about Evelyn. This demonstrates Lucretia's confused feelings of repressed sexuality: the desire for fulfillment through marriage and motherhood, mixed with a paralyzing fear of human contact that keeps her inside the apartment.

Lucretia's religious ties and her virginity, linked with her talk of "conception," also prompt Williams to ascribe to her the title of "madonna." We see the irony of this: she is not destined to become an adored maternal figure, but to spend the remainder of her life confined in an institution. Lucretia is a woman scorned by the man she loves. She lives alone, destitute and considered mad by those who know her.

What the others in the play say about her, and the attitudes they express about her condition and her fate provide a further understanding of the female madwoman. Except for the nurse, who appears at the end of the play, all the other characters are men; the two most prominent are the critical and unsympathetic elevator boy, Frank, and the understanding old porter, Nick; in these two figures we glimpse two common attitudes towards the mentally ill. Frank judges Lucretia harshly, calling her a "freak," "nuts," and insisting that she "don't have brain one." He wants to take some of her records for his girlfriend, but the porter insists that he not do so, for she "still got 'er property rights" (VI, 114). When Lucretia appears, Frank treats her rudely, sarcastically patronizing her and mocking her, although she is too distraught to notice. He finds her commentary of the rape "disgusting," and cannot contain his amusement when she claims to be pregnant.

Nick the porter, on the other hand, treats her with respect and understanding. He is the first to enter the apartment, and the stage directions describe his expression as one of "sorrowfully humorous curiosity" (VI, 110). When Frank calls Lucretia "nuts," Nick defends her, asserting that the world is full of strange people, many of them more dangerous than she. When Frank calls Lucretia "disgusting," Nick corrects him again, saying that she is pitiful, not disgusting. With Lucretia's appearance in the room, Nick takes on an attitude of politeness that demonstrates his compassion for her situation. Although both men humor her about her delusions, Nick does so in a way that does not belittle her; he is also very solicitous, helping her to the sofa and offering her his handkerchief when she begins to cry.

The two men's difference in age suggests that life experiences may influence the older man's attitude about those who suffer from mental illness. The younger man's demeanor is cocky and judgmental; he is quick to assume the worst about Lucretia, never considering how much she might be suffering. Nick, on the other hand, understands that human weakness comes in many forms. When he mentions all the other "maniacs" in Europe who should be confined, he implies that brutish behavior should be censored and punished, and harmless people like Lucretia should be left alone.

Later in the play, when Frank is taunting Lucretia, Nick tells the young man: "Cut that or git back in your cage" (VI, 118). With this command, Nick aligns the elevator boy with those brutish maniacs, thus reiterating his belief that those who commit acts of cruelty should be confined. This remark also suggests the lock-up of Miss Collins, who faces the "cage" of the asylum that awaits her, and at the end of the play, Williams makes this connection clear, when he notes in the stage directions that Lucretia disappears down the hall and the "elevator door clangs shut with the metallic sound of a locked cage" (VI, 126).

The other character from the apartment house, Mr. Abrams, the manager, expresses concern and compassion for Miss Collins; the stage directions tell us that he is "sincerely troubled by the situation" on the day that Lucretia faces institutionalization (VI, 124). The porter's statements about Mr. Abrams demonstrate that the latter is basically a good person, who has done what he could to care for Lucretia, managing her finances and securing a contribution from the church when her pension gave out. The present situation indicates that he can no longer make provisions for her to stay at the apartment house, and the elevator boy's comment about disturbing the neighbors suggests that Mr. Abrams has had some pressure put on him to evict Lucretia.

Although he is succumbing to that pressure, he also insists that Lucretia be treated with respect; when he brings the doctor and nurse to her apartment, he impresses upon the doctor that Miss Collins was "always a lady, Doctor, such a perfect lady" (VI, 125). When the nurse tries to hurry her along, Mr. Abrams insists that they not rush her, but allow her to finish the note she is writing to Richard. Once the group leaves for the hospital, the porter and Mr. Abrams read the note she left and briefly discuss what will become of Miss Collins's possessions. In their final exchange, the compassion that the two men feel is evident in their tones and in the way that they try to hide their feelings. The moment of awkwardness informs the audience that these men are genuinely sorry about what has happened, and yet they are not capable of making any other arrangements for Lucretia's future.

This ending is distinct from the later *Streetcar,* even though so many elements are similar. In *Streetcar,* Stella is sorry to see Blanche go, and she and Eunice try to calm Blanche's fears about her journey. The poker players rise as Blanche departs, signifying their respect for her, much the same way that the porter and Mr. Abrams allow Lucretia some dignity in her last moments of freedom. Once Blanche is gone, however, the conclusion of *Streetcar* focuses on the reunion of Stella and Stanley, with the appearance of their infant to complete the picture of family unity; this reunion is achieved at the cost of Blanche's freedom, and Stella's integrity.

The final scene of the longer play does not unambiguously settle what has happened in the apartment in Elysian Fields, but the struggle for supremacy between Blanche and Stanley is over, and Stanley has regained his position as head of household. *Madonna* is a slighter play, containing no parallel confrontation. The image we are left with, of two rather insignificant men who briefly defended the dignity of a delusional spinster, and then stay behind to clean up the mess she has left, makes for a poignant ending; this conclusion emphasizes the powerlessness of the madwoman, as well as the powerlessness of those who seek to protect her.

Madonna also reflects pointedly on the future of the madwoman in the asylum. Blanche's last words, spoken to the doctor in *Streetcar,* "Whoever you are—I have always depended on the kindness of strangers" (I, 418), suggest that the treatment Blanche will receive, from the doctor at least, will be more sympathetic than the treatment she has received from her relatives. The same cannot be assumed about Lucretia, for one gets the impression from her doctor and nurse that sympathy will not guide their behavior toward her. Rather, the respect Lucretia received from the porter and Mr. Abrams might be the last decent treatment she will ever receive. In both plays, however, the final scenes suggest a dismal future for these two women: bereft of choice, bereft of meaningful relationships, bereft of family ties.

Streetcar, first produced at the end of 1947, is notable in many ways, but surely one of the most enduring aspects of its success and acclaim is the manner in which it chronicles a woman's descent into madness. Blanche speaks of herself as ill in the opening scene of the play, but in scene two we get the first hint that eventually Stella and Stanley will join to put Blanche away; this is the initial sign of the danger that awaits Blanche. It is one thing for Blanche to call herself nervous and overwrought, and another for her relatives to speak in her absence about her condition. At the opening of scene two, Stanley enters to find Stella preparing to take Blanche out on the night of the poker game. When Stanley asks where his sister-in-law is, Stella replies that she is "soaking in a hot tub to quiet her nerves. She's terribly upset" (I, 269).

Thus, one day after Blanche arrives, we get our first glimpse of the couple's assessing Blanche's mental condition, with her out of earshot. Stella implores Stanley not to upset her sister, and particularly to say nothing about the loss of Belle Reve until Blanche is "calmed down"

(I, 271). Here we see a foreshadowing of the action that will dominate the last scene, when Blanche is removed to the institution against her will, without her knowledge. Early in the play, Stanley and Stella talk about Blanche and decide what is best for her. We also see that Stanley cares little about Blanche's nervous condition, while Stella seeks to protect Blanche, to do what is best for her.

This parallels the situation at the end of the play, for Stanley is equally unfeeling then about Blanche's commitment, and Stella still claims to be considering Blanche's best interest; at this point, however, it is clear to the audience that Stella seeks to save her marriage, thus agreeing to have Blanche committed because she cannot live with the reality of her sister's story of the rape.

The propensity for family members, often male, to arrange the commitment of female relatives, is noted by Yannick Ripa in her book *Women and Madness* (54-62). Although her book discusses nineteenth-century French women, many of her remarks present situations and attitudes appropriate to the time when Williams was writing. She notes that single women who were forced to work to support themselves were often more liable to be committed if they became unable to work. This is the situation Blanche faces at the opening of the play.

In scene seven, when Stanley tells Stella about what he has uncovered concerning Blanche's reputation in Laurel, he says that Blanche came to be regarded in her home town "as not just different but downright loco—nuts" (I, 361). Yet it is not until Blanche has been forced to resign her position as schoolteacher, and has come to reside in her sister's home, impoverished and without prospects for the future, that she is threatened with commitment. Ripa writes of the predicament of women who have no economic resources:

spinsters who became mentally ill became embarrassing—financially if their mental illness meant that they were not able to work, but also morally because their presence was a stain on the family, disturbed it with their symptoms and raised the constant problem of "dangerousness." . . . Nephews or brothers-in-law would therefore carry out the procedures necessary for commitment. (56)

In *Streetcar*, Blanche has come looking for asylum, and she has instead come to the place where she is most likely to end up in one. Recognition of the danger she faces as a penniless female suffering from nervous exhaustion is striking when Stanley and Stella first discuss her condition in scene two, but an exchange between Blanche and Stella in the opening scene foreshadows the conversation between the Kowalskis, especially in light of Ripa's remarks. When the sisters are talking about

Blanche staying at the apartment rather than at a hotel, Blanche's claim that she must stay with them and "can't be alone" prompts Stella to remark, "You seem a little bit nervous or overwrought or something." Blanche rather incongruously counters with a question, "Will Stanley like me, or will I be just a visiting in-law, Stella?" (I, 257). Thus we see that Blanche's nervousness about whether she has found a refuge, and her insecurity about whether her brother-in-law will endure her presence, highlight her precarious position in the Kowalski home.

Other similarities link scenes two and seven, and lead to a better understanding of the way that Stella and Stanley conspire against Blanche. Significantly, these are the only two scenes in the play where Stanley and Stella have opportunities for private discussion, and in both, Blanche's mental state and her future dominate the dialogue.

In both scenes, Blanche is taking a bath, singing songs in which she provides an unwitting commentary on her condition while Stanley and Stella discuss it. In scene two, she sings: "From the land of the sky blue water,/They brought a captive maid!" predicting her imminent captivity in the institution (I, 270). In addition, the "sky blue water" foreshadows her final long speech in the play, in which she speaks of dying at sea, her body "dropped overboard—at noon—in the blaze of summer—and into an ocean as blue as my first lover's eyes!" (I, 410). This connection is significant for a number of reasons, not only because madness is aligned with death, being a kind of death, a death of freedom, but also because Blanche's nervousness and instability are associated throughout the play with her marriage to the poet Allan Grey, the boy with those eyes.[6] So in her last speech of the play Blanche speaks of her death and her first lover, just before she is taken off to the asylum.

From the perspective of both stage reality and the dimensions of the Kowalski apartment, it is only while Blanche is in the bathroom that Stanley and Stella can speak privately, and only if she is singing and running water can they be certain to speak without her overhearing them. But Blanche singing of a "captive maid" while indulging in what she calls "hydrotherapy" at the same time that her sister and brother-in-law discuss her mental condition, comes down to more than just necessary staging; the scene forecasts what will happen later in the play.

In scene seven there are marked parallels to what the earlier scene introduced. Blanche is bathing again, and this time she is singing a song that includes the lyrics, "But it wouldn't be make-believe/If you believed in me!" At that time, Stanley is insuring that Stella no longer believes in her, as he has already done with Mitch (I, 360). At one point the stage directions indicate that in the bathroom "the water goes on loud; little breathless cries and peals of laughter are heard as if a child were frolicking in the tub" (I, 362). As in the earlier scene, Stanley and Stella discuss Blanche while she is unaware. This conversation is more ominous than the first because Stanley informs Stella about her sister's promiscuity, the reason Blanche departed from Laurel, and his plans to send her on a bus back to the town she has been asked to leave. Although Blanche never uses the ticket, it is significant that Stanley would fund her return, even though he knows she has been exiled from Laurel.

The final exchange between the two, before Blanche emerges from the bathroom, indicates that Stanley and Stella both realize that if Blanche cannot stay with them, and cannot return to her life in Laurel, something unmentionable awaits her in her future:

> Stella [slowly]: What'll-she-do? What on earth will she-do!
> Stanley: Her future is mapped out for her.
> Stella: What do you mean? (I, 367)

At that point Stanley breaks off their conversation and calls for Blanche to get out of the bathroom. He does not answer his wife's question, and therefore leaves us wondering just what he thinks Blanche's future will contain. Although he is not specific, this exchange signals what is to come, for it is the Kowalskis who decide Blanche's fate, not Blanche herself. Her singing and giggling in the tub throughout this scene reveal how far she is from knowing what is being decided about her in the other room; however, the stage directions indicate that she registers fear, "almost a look of panic," when she does emerge from her bath, her hydrotherapy.

Besides the information these two scenes give us about how her relatives will decide what is to become of her, both of these private talks between Stanley and Stella center on Blanche's economic condition, a condition inextricably tied to her family's power to decide her future. In scene two we discover that Blanche has lost the family home, Belle Reve, and so her situation is not only one of a woman suffering from nervous exhaustion, who has lost her income, it is of one who has also lost the place where she might have been able to shield herself from the censure of the community. The people of Laurel still might have regarded her as "downright loco—nuts," as Stanley puts it, but had she a place to live without danger of eviction, she might have remained in her hometown.

By coming to New Orleans and placing herself at the mercy of her relatives, admitting that she has lost Belle Reve, Blanche becomes economically vulnerable to Stanley's plans to extricate her from the apartment. This tie between economic dependence and the ability for others to commit her against her will becomes more strikingly apparent in scene seven, when Stanley emphasizes her joblessness—"She's not going back to teach school!" (I, 362); her homelessness—"They told her she better move on to some fresh territory" (I, 363); and his decision to expel her from the premises—"She's not staying here after Tuesday" (I, 367).

Most critics have viewed Blanche's rootlessness as an aspect of her role as a faded southern belle. Lindy Melman, for example, insists that her homelessness "goes far deeper than the simple fact that she has no roof over her head. She is an anachronism, forced to live in a world that has discarded all adherence to her particular tradition" (126). While Melman is correct in focusing on Blanche's inability to leave behind her the tradition of the Old South, and embrace the new world order represented by Stanley, as her sister has done, this explanation for Blanche's fate does not consider her mental condition, or how that condition directs her fate.

That fate is sealed when Stanley rapes her, but her mental instability is clear throughout the play, and from the opening scene Williams stresses her nervousness and her fragile mental condition. When she is alone in the apartment in the first scene, waiting for Stella to come she tells herself: "I've got to keep hold of myself!" (I, 250). Then, when Stella arrives and offers her a mixed drink with coke, she responds, "No coke, honey, not with my nerves tonight!" (I, 251). Filling Stella in on why she has appeared before the school term ended, she informs her sister that her nerves broke, and she "was on the verge of—lunacy, almost!" (I, 254).

These remarks are just the beginning of Blanche's litany of self-revealing comments, for she seems to recognize how close she is to the edge of insanity. In scene six she insists to Mitch that "a single girl, a girl alone in the world, has got to keep a firm hold on her emotions or she'll be lost!" (I, 343). Although in the immediate context she is speaking of her romantic involvement with Mitch, in the larger view of the play and considering the precariousness of the single woman's role in society, her remark resonates with the implication that if she does not remain emotionally fit, she will become one of the lost women who ends up institutionalized. While in the last scene Blanche seems unaware of her fate, she gives numerous indications throughout the rest of the play that she recognizes her frail mental condition, and the consequences of that condition if she gets pushed toward the brink of insanity.

To add to the effect of her words, Williams uses "hysterically" and "nervously" in his stage directions throughout the play, signaling that the actress should take care to appear on the edge of collapse. This is not to say that the audience or reader does not witness a decline in Blanche's stability—she drinks more as the play proceeds, and is "boxed out of her mind" during scenes nine and ten, when Mitch comes to see her, and when Stanley finally returns from the hospital. In the early scenes Blanche reverts to calm behavior, but she loses this ability as the action proceeds.

That she can still hold her own in a contest of wills becomes especially evident during the latter half of scene two, when Blanche and Stanley discuss Belle Reve and the "Napoleonic code." Blanche's strength at this point in the play is outlined very well by Anca Vlasopolos in her article on the struggle between the two characters over the different versions of history they represent. The critic rightly indicates early in her examination of the play that the "ultimate measure of the struggle represented in *A Streetcar Named Desire* is the opposition of reason to unreason, of sanity to lunacy" (Vlasopolos 152). Vlasopolos's discussion precedes my own preoccupation with the theme of madness, and in her explication of scene two, in connection with her own thesis, she argues that Stanley represents the patriarchy, an argument aligned with my theory that Blanche's defeat is in part due to her powerlessness in the society.

In scene two, however, Blanche has not yet succumbed to the forces of authority, and she resists Stanley's efforts to bully her into submission. Vlasopolos argues that in this scene Stanley's "authority is undercut by his obvious and avowed ignorance of anything outside the immediate sphere of his experience," citing as evidence Stanley's repeated mention of "acquaintances" who will apprise him of the worth of Blanche's furs and jewels, as well as the legal status of the estate (155). Although she is correct in noting that Stanley wrongly assumes that Blanche's things are valuable, and that false bravado lies at the root of his remarks on the "Napoleonic code," Stanley's comic reference to authority figures turns to tragedy when "authorities" from the asylum take Blanche away.

Nonetheless, Blanche is not beaten in this early scene, and Vlasopolos points out that having begun the scene "as a stranger who is being discussed behind her back and whose possessions are being rifled for a clue about her criminality, Blanche rises in scene two to a position of authority vis-à-vis both Stella and Stanley" (155). Blanche's collapse has not yet occurred, and it is useful to compare this Blanche to the woman of the final scene to become cognizant of the deterioration the play dramatizes. Despite her nervousness throughout the play, and her frequent references to her emotional precariousness, Blanche can still rise to defend herself verbally, and thus fend off her attackers when she senses danger. When she loses this ability, the Kowalskis attain power over her fate.

One important aspect of her defense is her class superiority over Stanley. While Vlasopolos's essay places Stanley firmly within the power position, a representative of the patriarchy, Blanche's strength in the play's early scenes depends upon her awareness that Stanley is lower-class, a "different species" (I, 258). Pointing out his crudeness to Stella continually, Blanche forces her sister into temporary alliances against Stanley. This struggle reaches a climax in scene eight, during the birthday celebration, when Stella's complaints about Stanley's table manners result in his outburst:

Don't ever talk that way to me! "Pig—Polack—disgusting—vulgar—greasy!" —them kind of words have been on your tongue and your sister's too much around here! What do you two think you are? A pair of queens? (I, 371)

His rage, which he expresses by throwing dishes to the floor, suggests that he recognizes the truth in their words; this scene demonstrates his frustration and defensiveness, and results in a measure of sympathy for Stanley. Blanche has, after all, launched constant attacks against her brother-in-law, and seeks to turn Stella against him.

Stanley's ultimate victory, however, is suggested by his remark immediately following his suggestion that the two women think they are queens: "Remember what Huey Long said—'Every Man is a King!' And I am the king around here, so don't forget it!" (I, 371). The statement implies his recognition that despite his lower-class status, his maleness ensures his dominance. Later in the scene, he elaborates on his control over Stella:

When we first met, me and you, you thought I was common. How right you was, baby. I was common as dirt. You showed me the snapshot of the place with the columns. I pulled you down off them columns and how you loved it, having them colored lights going! (I, 377)

He acknowledges that his power over her is sexual, even rather violent ("I pulled you down"); his attitude towards sexual power leads him to rape Blanche in order to control her. In both cases, his sexual potency proves stronger than the women's claims to class superiority, for Stanley possesses the "power and pride of a richly feathered male bird among hens" (I, 265).

Blanche's expectations of survival are not pinned solely on her attempts to turn Stella against Stanley. Until scene seven, the prospect that Mitch will provide sanctuary for Blanche, "a cleft in the rock of the world that I could hide in," mediates the hopelessness of her situation; if Mitch marries her, she "can leave here and not be anyone's problem" (I, 335). Significantly, in order for Mitch to accept her, she feels she must appear chaste. In his final rejection of her, he makes it clear that he cannot accept her past sexual exploits, and that she is "not clean enough to bring in the house with my mother" (I, 390). Blanche's promiscuity has been the subject of much critical discussion of her predicament, but her sexual activity not only causes Mitch to reject her, it establishes her as a prime candidate for an asylum. Ever since the Greeks mistakenly associated hysteria with a disorder of the womb, female sexuality and insanity have been linked by theories of cause and effect.

As Elaine Showalter discusses in *The Female Malady,* Victorian psychiatry defined its role in managing women in part as "the enforcement in the asylum of those qualities of self-government and industriousness that would help a woman resist the stresses of her body and the weaknesses of her female nature." She adds that "uncontrolled sexuality seemed the major, almost defining symptom of insanity in women" (74).

Similarly, in speaking of the efforts to repress sexuality in the asylum, Yannick Ripa claims that medicine saw "hysterical women, nymphomaniacs and erotomaniacs . . . as sexual deviations and as pathological phenomena" (132). Both write of the use of clitoral amputation as a "cure" for promiscuity within the asylum, and Ripa also mentions the use of hydrotherapy to control sexual impulses (significantly, this is Blanche's practice and even the term she uses for her hot baths). The connection between sexuality and madness does not disappear with the end of the nineteenth century, however, and Phyllis Chesler, in her study of women and madness in 1970s United States, remarks that women "have already been bitterly and totally repressed sexually; many may be reacting to or trying to escape from just such repression, and the powerlessness it signifies, by 'going mad'" (37).

Another indication that Mitch provides a possibility of salvation for Blanche is that the Varsouviana, the polka tune that Blanche associates with her husband's suicide, that plays in her head when she is upset, is a central feature of her two major scenes with Mitch. In scene six, when Blanche confides in Mitch the details of Allan Grey's death, the polka music dies out when Mitch embraces her. Thus, Mitch represents a hope that security in marriage would terminate the hauntings of the past that plague Blanche and intensify her hysteria.

At the opening of scene nine, when Mitch arrives to confront her about her past, the stage directions indicate that the Varsouviana is playing, and that it is "in her mind; she is drinking to escape it and the sense of disaster closing in on her" (I, 379). This time, Mitch's words are not comforting to her, and the polka tune stops only when she hears the shot. With Mitch's rejection, Blanche's hope for salvation is extinguished, and the polka tune is a prologue to the lurid reflections and the overwhelming music of the next scene, the final confrontation with Stanley.

Stanley's rape of Blanche in scene ten occurs while Stella spends the night at the hospital, delivering their baby. This plot device provides the opportunity for Stanley and Blanche to be alone together, thus facilitating the rape. That the rape occurs while Stella delivers the baby also points up the marked contrast between Blanche's sexuality and Stella's: Stella's sexual encounters with Stanley produce a baby; Blanche's sexual encounter with Stanley results in her madness. Besides embracing Stanley's lifestyle and values in order to escape the death and decay of Belle Reve, Stella has welcomed the sexual role of the happily married woman —she adores her husband, and seems eager to bear him children. From the opening scene, she makes it clear to Blanche that her sexual life with Stanley is exciting and satisfying. Louise Blackwell, in her study of Williams's women, defines Stella as one of Williams's women "who have subordinated themselves to a domineering and often inferior person to attain reality and meaning through communication with another person" (102).

In scene four, in the aftermath of the poker night, even though her husband struck her in a drunken rage, Stella has reconciled with him and lies in a state of "narcotized tranquility" in the aftermath of their lovemaking. On the other hand, Blanche is frantic about the previous evening's events; she "has spent a sleepless night and her appearance entirely contrasts with Stella's" (I, 310). Throughout this scene she is nervous and emotional, insisting that Stella face up to her situation, and escape from Stanley with her. Stella has no intention of doing so, and it is clear that her night with Stanley has erased any anxiety she may have felt about his brutality. Stanley and Stella's sexual relations bolster their marital relations, and Stella's emotional state is tranquil.

Conversely, a violent sexual encounter between Blanche and Stanley drives her over the brink of insanity. Unlike Stella, Blanche has not found fulfillment or tranquillity in sexual encounters; ever since her unsatisfactory marriage to Allan Grey, who preferred men, her experience has been confined to "intimacies with strangers." While some of those intimacies were with inappropriate companions (particularly in the case of her young student), the condemnation she receives from Mitch and from Stanley seems to be unspecific, not clearly restricted to her inappropriate couplings. Stanley's words to her just before he rapes her, "We've had this date with each other from the beginning," implies that he is not raping her because he now knows of her sexual promiscuity, but because she is single and comes to stay with him and Stella (I, 402).[7] Since the rape precipitates her madness, and it occurs while Stella fulfills one of her most important wifely duties, the rape stands as a representation of Blanche's inability to conform to the sexual standards for women in her society, and she is punished for that shortcoming.

Blanche's expulsion from the society of the Quarter at the end of the play not only results from Stella's decision to stand by her husband and "deny" the rape; it also hinges on the fact that Mitch's rejection and Stanley's hostility leave Blanche no other options. Her commitment results from the need for a woman in this society to have a secure place: she has confused her departure with the rescue by Shep Huntleigh that she has spoken of and wished for throughout the play, thus emphasizing the necessity of a male savior.

When the doctor and nurse arrive, Blanche is upset by the nurse's presence, and refuses to accompany her, but she willingly leaves with the doctor, even though she realizes that he is not the gentleman she was expecting. Blanche, "holding tight to his arm" and allowing him "to lead her as if she were blind," departs from the scene in the company of the only man who will accept and care for her—the hospital psychiatrist. Blanche's descent into madness has been inextricably tied to her impoverished single status, her subsequent search for male protection, and her refusal to accept the restrictive sexual norms prescribed for women. Although this pattern is repeated in other Williams plays and in other of Williams characters, Blanche stands as the supreme example of how the playwright dramatizes the intersection of women and madness. Nowhere else does he succeed in balancing the madwoman's culpability and vulnerability in such equal proportions.

In *Suddenly Last Summer* (1958), the woman confined for madness is not middle-aged, and although she is unmarried, she does not fit the profile of a spinster so often designated as stereotypically Williams. The Doctor and Mrs. Venable speak of her as a girl, and although we are not sure of her age, she is attractive, for she tells the doctor that Sebastian used her to procure men for him. Yet some aspects of Catharine Holly's predicament are comparable with those of Blanche and Lucretia: her economic plight, and the ways that others in the play, especially her family members, speak of her and treat her as if she cannot decide her own future.

The question of Catharine's sanity hinges on the truth or falsity of the story she has told about the murder of her cousin, Sebastian. She accompanied him on his annual trip, and he was killed while they were in Mexico. Catharine's account of his death is a horrid tale of human cannibalism; since telling this story she has been locked up in a private asylum, her care paid for by Violet Venable, Catharine's aunt and Sebastian's mother.

When the play opens, Mrs. Venable has arranged for a doctor from the state institution to examine Catharine in order to determine if she is an eligible candidate for the experimental lobotomy treatment he has developed. The opening scene establishes Violet's adoration of her son, and her desperate insistence on protecting his reputation, which she feels has been slandered by Catharine's tale of his death. The lobotomy would solve Violet's problem, for she feels that it would "cut" the story out of her niece's brain; even when the doctor points out that it might not do so, Violet is secure in the fact that "after the operation, who would believe her, Doctor?" (III, 367).

In this first scene we also learn that Violet and Sebastian supported Catharine, for Violet tells the doctor that they "put the bread in her mouth and the clothes on her back" (III, 363). Indeed, Violet feels that Catharine's dependence causes the girl to resent her aunt and cousin, and Violet insists that this resentment drives Catharine to fabricate the story of Sebastian's horrific death.

Since Violet has also supported Catharine's mother and brother, the Holly family abides by Violet's wishes to confine Catharine to a private mental institution. Violet expresses her contempt for the Hollys in remarking to the doctor, "These people are not blood relatives of mine, they're my dead husband's relations. I always detested these people, my dead husband's sister and—her two worthless children" (III, 391). But Violet also makes it clear that she begrudgingly provided for them financially, "doing more than my duty to keep their heads above water" (III, 391). She explains that her son, Sebastian, insisted on it, "being excessively softhearted." In a position of financial dependence, the Hollys are anxious to keep Violet happy, for Sebastian has named the Holly children in his will, and if Violet chooses to contest it, they will be without income. Now that Sebastian is dead, Violet will no longer feel compelled to support them.

Thus, Catharine's wild story about Sebastian's death, that he was eaten alive by beggar children, makes the Holly family, and most especially Catharine, extremely vulnerable to Violet's anger. The Hollys are convinced, quite rightly, that as long as Catharine insists on telling that story, Violet will contest the will and tie the money up indefinitely. Mrs. Venable cannot accept the gruesomeness of Catharine's story; she also resents Catharine because Sebastian decided to take Catharine with him to Europe rather than her. Catharine tells the doctor that Violet's slight stroke "was disfiguring, and after that, Sebastian couldn't use her"

(III, 396). Thus, Catharine replaced Violet in the role of sexual procurer; to Violet, this means Catharine became more important to Sebastian, and this alone is sufficient reason for Violet to despise Catharine.

When Sebastian died, and Catharine related the circumstances of his death, Violet released her anger and frustration by committing her niece to St. Mary's, and now intends to silence her once and for all by arranging for the lobotomy. Catharine's story is difficult to accept, and provides reason enough for the authorities to question the girl's sanity. Everything that Violet says about Sebastian indicates that she judges his life by standards she would not impose on anyone else. Violet cannot believe that he would seek out the company of beggars, or in any way put himself in a position in which he might be vulnerable to them. Violet's speeches convince us that she holds her son in the highest regard; however, when Catharine arrives, and provides details of this family's life, we can no longer be sure that Violet's motives are entirely prompted by her need to protect her son's name.

Apart from the resentment Violet bears Catharine for replacing her, Mrs. Venable's description of Catharine's social debut indicates that removing Catharine from society would free the family from disgrace. Violet informs the doctor that no one liked Catharine, although she does admit "She had some kind of—notoriety! She had a sharp tongue that some people mistook for wit. A habit of laughing in the faces of decent people which would infuriate them, and also reflected adversely on me and Sebastian, too" (III, 391). Although she admits that her son was amused by Catharine, Violet herself was "disgusted, sickened."

Violet had reasons, therefore, for wanting Catharine silenced before Sebastian took her with him on the fateful trip. Her final outburst in the play, when she screams for the doctor to "cut this hideous story out of her brain," suggests that she wants her "sharp tongue" silenced (III, 423). Other talk of the way Catharine "babbles" and the way the operation "quiets them down," although referring to Violet's wish to suppress the story of Sebastian's murder, might also indicate that Catherine has always caused embarrassment to the family, and that Violet is now taking the opportunity to rid herself of a nuisance she has always endured.

Another story that Catharine tells the doctor provides further evidence of Catherine's inability to maintain propriety about unmentionable things. Violet alludes to the circumstances of this story when she tells the doctor that Catharine was dropped from the New Orleans social set when "she'd lost her head over a young married man, made a scandalous scene at a Mardi Gras ball, in the middle of the ballroom" (III, 392). Catharine gives us more details, explaining how a married man lured her away from the ball, made love to her in the woods, then took her home, telling her to forget him because his wife was pregnant. This incident aligns Catharine with the other women of this chapter, since the episode is an unfortunate sexual alliance with an unavailable man, and the incident seems to have the same kind of effect on Catharine that similar incidents have on Blanche and Lucretia. Blanche's unhappy marriage to Allan, who, because of his homosexuality is emotionally and physically unavailable to his wife, causes her to strike out against him and instigate his suicide. His death ends any happiness in her life, for when he shoots himself "the searchlight which had been turned on the world was turned off again and never for one moment since has there been any light that's stronger than this—kitchen—candle" (I, 355).

The incident in *Suddenly Last Summer* also takes place at a dance, and creates a stir among the guests. After the man drops her off and tells her to forget him, Catharine returns to the ballroom, intending to retrieve the coat she borrowed from Violet. She sees the man who has just seduced her: "I ran up to him and beat him as hard as I could in the face and chest with my fists" (III, 399). Like Blanche, Catharine feels compelled to punish the man who has so cruelly used and betrayed her, and like Blanche, this incident seems to bring a change in her life: "[T]he next morning, I started writing my diary in the third person, singular," and "I couldn't go out any more" (III, 399). Soon after this development, Sebastian decides to have her accompany him on his trip; thus, the incident at the dance begins a new phase in Catharine's life.

Since the man was married and his wife pregnant, her feelings that he betrayed her suggest a similarity between Catharine and Lucretia; for both of them, having feelings for a man who cannot reciprocate, feelings that are improper in light of the circumstances, helps to provide the opportunity for other people to have them institutionalized. In Catharine's case, her feelings seem to transfer from this man to her cousin Sebastian, and this proves to be another inappropriate alliance, for not only is Sebastian homosexual, he is a close blood relative. In the climatic scene of the play, when Catharine is about to tell her story for the doctor, Violet suggests that Catherine did have romantic feelings for Sebastian, crying out, "She was in love with my son!" (III, 392).

These women characters choose to indulge in relationships (in Lucretia's case the relationship is imaginary) that are inappropriate or impossible, and because of these relationships, their sanity is questioned. In *Suddenly*, a woman relative arranges for the commitment, a circumstance that demonstrates that Williams does not propose that only men wield the power to have others silenced in this manner. Although all the plays cause us to consider whether institutionalization is necessary or appropriate, *Suddenly* does not clearly establish Catharine's behavior as unusual. The question of Catharine's sanity has been debated by critics of the play, who have suggested a number of possible outcomes for the play's conclusion, indicating that Williams leaves the ending ambiguous.[8]

Catharine has suffered from depression, and after the incident at the ball, refuses to leave the house. Also, she begins to write her diary in the third person, and this expresses a feeling of separation from the self, a common symptom of schizophrenia. However, when she speaks of this time to the doctor, she speaks lucidly of this feeling within her, and since she no longer speaks of herself in the third person, her madness does not lie there.

At the opening of scene two, when Catharine first arrives at the Venable home, the nun who accompanies her indicates that Catharine has been unmanageable, and her attitude toward Catharine suggests that she does think the girl is mentally ill. The sister refuses to let the girl smoke, even when Catharine points out that she is away from the hospital and might depart from the rules without penalty. The nun tries to persuade Catharine to give her the lighted cigarette, as if she thinks Catharine is dangerous; Catharine defends herself against these charges in a rational way. Catharine explains that her smoking privileges were rescinded because she burned a hole in her skirt, and she maintains that this happened because she was "half unconscious under medication" (III, 371). When the sister still refuses to allow her to smoke, and insists that Catharine hand over the cigarette, Catharine does so by thrusting the lighted end of the cigarette into the nun's hand.

While this does seem violent, Catharine explains herself by declaring: "I'm sick, I'm sick—of being bossed and bullied!" (III, 372). This episode convinces us that the nun could have avoided the situation by allowing the girl to smoke. Catharine's defense of her action suggests not insanity but anger at the treatment she receives.

Most of Catharine's behavior reflects clear thinking and an acute awareness of her condition and her possible fate. She knows about Lion's View state hospital and the experimental surgery that the doctor has been performing there. When her brother and mother speak with her privately, Catharine exhibits complete cognizance, even explaining to her family that if the doctor gives her an injection she will not be able to adjust her story to please them, but will be forced to tell the truth, however horrible that may be. Her brother George concludes that she knows exactly what she is doing, that she is "crazy like a coyote," and that she is "no more crazy than I am, she's just, just—PERVERSE! Was ALWAYS!— perverse" (III, 381-82). George's conclusion stems from his anger and frustration at the possibility that he will lose his inheritance because of Catharine, but his choice of words to describe his sister suggests that her insistence on straying from the norms of polite behavior rather than any diagnosis of madness may be the reason she is now confined .

Deciding whether Catharine is sane must take into account her story, which is her aunt's primary reason for having her locked up. We cannot be sure if the description that Catharine gives of Sebastian's death is accurate, for the play does not offer any corroboration of her story in the form of other witnesses. Surely the most horrifying and unbelievable part of the story is that the beggar children ate the parts of Sebastian that they tore away from his body with their "instruments." As Ruby Cohn points out, even if we assume that Catharine is telling what she thinks is the truth, she did not witness the murder itself (she ran away down the hill) but only its aftermath, so she cannot say with certainty that the children actually ate Sebastian, but only that they tore his body apart (Cohn, *Dialogue* 117). From this perspective, then, we realize that we cannot determine whether or not Catharine's story is true, and hence, if she is insane.

On the other hand, her story seems believable because of what we learn about Sebastian and his life, especially from Violet. The Venus flytrap in the Venable garden, and the flesh-eating birds of the Encantadas both foreshadow the story of the beggars devouring Sebastian, and therefore lend it credence. When Violet can so easily accept the dark side of Sebastian's inquiry into the nature of god, and yet cannot accept that he could himself be consumed by such a force, it leads us to consider that Violet may be trying to rid herself of Catharine for other reasons.

Whatever those reasons are, her refusal to believe Catharine's story parallels Stella's refusal to believe Blanche's story about the rape in *Streetcar*. Even though Violet's disbelief is more calculated and diabolical, especially considering that she is willing to ensure the lobotomy by offering the doctor money, both Violet and Stella choose to sacrifice the female who threatens them, in order to preserve the reputation of the male. Stella also wants to protect her marriage, her own future and her baby's future. In both cases, the threats to Blanche and Catharine are to their sanity, and therefore to their freedom. These women face permanent institutionalization as a direct result of the men with whom they became involved. Even though there is no indication that Sebastian and Catharine had a sexual relationship, he used her to establish power for himself, much as Stanley used Blanche to assert his power within the family. Stanley and Sebastian come to different ends, to be sure, since Sebastian is himself a sacrifice, but he sets Catharine up for the danger she faces, just as surely as Stanley sets up Blanche.

The character most sympathetic to Catharine's story turns out to be her brother, who has never thought that she was crazy, but was the least pleased with her insistence on telling the tale of Sebastian's death. When Catharine finishes telling the group what happened to Sebastian, Violet reacts by attempting to strike Catharine, and then, as she is led away, calls for her destruction, for the doctor to "cut this hideous story out of her brain!"; at this, George speaks up and tells his mother that he will quit school and get a job (III, 423). Originally quite concerned about his inheritance, George now contends that he will free the family of Violet's stranglehold by supporting them himself. Since the doctor's suggestion that Catharine's story "could be true," follows this turnaround by George, we are led to believe her story has convinced them. Presumably, the doctor will not allow the operation, and Catharine will be released. But the truth or falsehood of the story Catharine tells of human cannibalism cannot be determined, and perhaps the horror of the story only suggests that when the truth is too horrible, the tendency is to free oneself from it. If this freedom involves locking someone else away, so be it.

Williams's late play *Clothes for a Summer Hotel,* first performed in 1980, also deals with madness, and provides an interesting departure from these earlier works in a number of notable ways. Of the plays I have discussed thus far, *Clothes* is the only one whose setting is a mental institution, and the play's central action concerns a husband's visit to his wife at this asylum. The couple are real-life figures, F. Scott and Zelda Fitzgerald.[9] Throughout the play, male and female are compared and contrasted, and the gender issue is a prominent factor in our understanding of the characters and the action.

This play resembles the earlier ones in its focus on female insanity, but since the play is set in the institution, the conflict does not center on the possibility of commitment: for Zelda, commitment is already a reality. Scott is visiting his wife at the asylum where she is confined, and the action slips back and forth from present to past, with no clear indication of when the present actually is. Early in the play, when the intern is encouraging Zelda to go outside to see Scott, she resists, remarking: "I thought that obligations stopped with death"; this implies that she has died already and that the action takes place after death (*Clothes* 8).

In keeping with Zelda's comment, Williams calls the play a ghost play, suggesting that the characters are ghosts of what they were in life, and that the action consists of memories, therefore fallible. Williams also states in his author's note that "in a sense all plays are ghost plays, since players are not actually whom they play." He goes on to explain that taking liberty with time and place is fitting with what occurs on the grounds of a asylum, "where liberties of this kind are quite prevalent," and "these liberties allow us to explore in more depth what we believe is truth of character" (Author's Note).

This ambiguity might be intended to soften the fact of Zelda's commitment, for the suggestion that the events of the play are memories makes the reality of the institution easier to accept. On the other hand, however, the asylum setting dominates the stage, with a mock-up of the asylum building, and, more important, "a pair of Gothic-looking black gates, rather unrealistically tall" (note on the set). In a way, Williams has thus captured the paradox of asylum life: the inmates exist in a setting removed from time and place, where they often create their own particular version of reality with hallucinations and delusions. Simultaneously, the setting in which they live is one of implacable concreteness: stone or brick buildings, barred windows, locked doors and gates. Zelda's character in the play is at times caught up in memories of the past, at times frustrated by the limitations of the rules of asylum life, and forced to face the husband who has traveled to visit her after a long separation between them.

Unlike the other women characters I have studied in this chapter, Zelda is not a spinster, but the wife of one of the most celebrated writers of this century. She has lived a legendary life, but has ended up in an asylum for the mentally ill. Her husband has just arrived from Hollywood to see her, having been mistakenly informed that she is much improved. When she sees him, Zelda remarks on his life in Hollywood: "Isn't it sort of a madhouse, too? You occupy one there, and I occupy one here" (12). Throughout the play, Scott, Zelda and the other characters compare the husband and wife to each other, and their intertwined lives, as well as their different fates, allow Williams to suggest how gender affects one's life choices and options.

Scott's "madhouse" does not have a locked gate, or nuns who pose as guards; despite the suggestions that both suffer imprisonment, Zelda's confinement contains insulin treatments. She refers to it as "torture," but Scott insists that she is not forced to stay. She defends her return there from visits to her mother, insisting that she comes back to escape the reactions people have to her outside the asylum: she is "pointed out on the street as a lunatic now" (13). Scott argues that whatever the reason, "you do return by choice, so don't call it confinement" (13). The husband feels it necessary to convince his wife that she has chosen her residence since this choice would absolve him of guilt or responsibility.

Scott's visit upsets Zelda, and the intern (who is alternately Edouard, Zelda's French lover) complains to the doctor that Scott "has disturbed his wife" (19). Shortly after this, when Scott claims that he will not leave until "discovering who's responsible for my wife's condition," Edouard replies, "And if you learn it is you?" (21). Williams implicates Scott when exploring the causes of Zelda's disturbed condition.

Zelda alternates between blaming herself for Scott's shortcomings, and blaming him for her madness. Early in the play, she implies that they both used each other: "I have the eyes of a hawk which is a bird of nature as predatory as a husband who appropriates your life as material for his writing" (12). She goes on to say that had he considered her predatory nature before marrying her, he could have been saved completely for his art. Thus, she acknowledges that she has interfered with his writing, that perhaps he would have been a better writer without having to worry about her. Zelda makes this more explicit when she says that he was not to blame for their failures, for, she tells him: "You needed a better influence, someone much more stable as a companion on the—roller-coaster ride which collapsed at the peak" (15). She does not say exactly what these failures are, but implies that they include her madness and his drinking.

Scott blames her for disrupting his life with her emotional problems, telling the intern: "I've sold, am selling my talent, bartering my life and my daughter's future in the obviously vain hope that—here at Highland you could—return her to—" (22). When the intern asks him to what Zelda should return, Scott screams, "REASON, REASON, GOD DAMN IT!" Scott holds Zelda and her insanity responsible for forcing him to be a commercial success, perhaps indicating that this need interferes with his creative freedom. Since he is living and writing in Hollywood at the time, he may be sacrificing his artistic freedom to make money by writing for the movies.[10] Scott supports Zelda, and speaks of it more than once, indicating that Zelda is as impoverished as the other madwomen in this chapter; even though she has a certain amount of security in having a husband, she is as financially dependent on him as Catharine is on Violet, as Blanche is on Stanley and Stella, and as Lucretia is on the charity of the church.

Scott's accusations towards Zelda, however, are not as significant or believable as those that Zelda makes against Scott: that she has sacrificed her life and her sanity for his art. This accusation constitutes the major conflict of the play, and is central to any understanding of how madness works as a major theme. When Zelda tells Scott that she has taken up ballet in the asylum, as a form of occupational therapy, she insists that dance has become the "career that I undertook because you forbade me to write" (13). She is too old to dance, and her figure is bloated from the insulin treatment she has received, so pursuing ballet at this time in her life is an indication that she has lost touch with reality.

More significant than this, however, is her suggestion that her writing talents have been suppressed by Scott, and that he has no interest in helping her to realize her literary ambitions. In Act 1, scene 2, during a flashback to about 1926, Scott accuses Zelda of interrupting his work, and she in turn says: "What about my work?" (33). When, a few moments later she repeats her question, having received no satisfactory response from him, he makes it clear to her that he considers her work to be "the work that all Southern ladies dream of performing some day. Living well with a devoted husband and child" (36). Scott implies that this role should be the only one that she should aspire to, but Zelda responds to this assertion: "Sorry, wrong size, it pinches!—Can't wear that shoe, too confining" (36). Zelda's situation is quite different, therefore, than that of the women in the earlier plays: she has the married life that they do not, and yet this life has not proved fulfilling, and has not protected her from insanity. Perhaps the suggestion is that when these women are unable to secure for themselves the kind of life they desire, whether it be as wife or mother or writer, the confining nature of the life they must settle for instead is what drives them into madness.

Zelda's predicament recalls the argument Louise Blackwell made about the major female characters of the earlier plays: that they sought a mate and therefore a sexually secure and stable life. Zelda has secured a mate, and yet she is not fulfilled; in fact, one incident from her past that is dramatized in *Clothes* is her affair with a French aviator, when marriage to Scott became unsatisfying. This situation suggests that marriage does not provide the emotional security Zelda needs, but her affair also qualifies her as another promiscuous madwoman.

Although Scott suffers from alcoholism, drinking to alleviate anxiety, a trademark of the nervous types Williams protrays, it does not threaten his sanity. The implication that Scott's work saves him from similar long term institutionalization makes Zelda's case more poignant, for she seeks artistic outlets as well, but cannot escape the asylum. Her ballet dancing, instead of acting as an artistic release, convinces others of her madness. Zelda sums up her life, and indeed all life, as an attempt to escape the kind of confinement that she has spoken of, claiming: "Between the first wail of an infant and the last gasp of the dying—it's all an arranged pattern of—submission to what's been prescribed for us unless we escape into madness or acts of creation" (71). Scott's insistence on suppressing her work confines Zelda and forces her into the only other path of escape she recognizes: the path to the asylum, and to another kind of confinement. Whether or not Scott is to blame is debatable, but Zelda is not the only character in the play who makes this claim. Gerald Murphy and one of Zelda's psychiatrists both comment on the high quality of Zelda's writing, and in both cases Scott reacts defensively to their claims that he selfishly protected his own interests as a writer at the expense of her talents. Their opinions strengthen Zelda's case against Scott.

Clothes delves into the question of Fitzgerald's sexuality, offering a scene between him and Hemingway that suggests both men's sexual ambiguity; Scott and Zelda's relationship, however, remains the most developed issue in the play. Although the time and place of the action shifts from the asylum to times and places in the Fitzgeralds' past, the iron gates dominate the stage throughout the play, and the reality of Zelda's institutionalization is never far from the center of the action. The nuns who guard the gates, the intern who guides Zelda, and the doctors who consult with Scott are the visual reminders that this play, like the ones discussed earlier, focus on a woman whose life story includes the barred window, the straitjacket, and the locked gate.

Tennessee Williams's women characters often survive tragedy or loss, witness the unspeakable, and face unbearable loneliness; the plays I have discussed capture the essence of their suffering by dramatizing the moments at which they can no longer fight to survive in a cruel world. When they reach this breaking point, although they may consider suicide, they cannot choose it. But they do often die in another way: they escape into madness.

Invariably, this madness comes upon them when they are most emotionally vulnerable, but also when they are economically vulnerable and displaced from society's approved ways of life. Because of society's conventions and restrictions on women, they are frequently unable to make the choices that might ensure emotional stability, or at least safety from those who wish to silence their protests and accusations. In Williams's plays, the attempts to silence and control these women does not result in death, but in institutionalization.

3

Babbling Lunatics: Language and Madness

Tell all the Truth but tell it slant—
—Emily Dickinson

Lion's View! State asylum, cut this hideous story out of her brain!
—Violet in *Suddenly Last Summer*

The final exit of Blanche DuBois in the celebrated original production of *A Streetcar Named Desire* on Broadway was a familiar image to Americans of the late 1940s: not only to those who saw that first production but to anyone who read about the play in newspapers or magazines. Blanche's departure on the doctor's arm, depending on his kindness, his gallantry contrasted with the severity of the matron, was reproduced in many articles and reviews about the play and its playwright. A number of factors make this an excellent choice for publicity: all the principals are present, along with the important supporting players; the still makes excellent use of the features of the set, with its interior/exterior design, for we are able to see Blanche departing as well as the card game inside the flat; Stanley and Stella's reconciliation scene occupies the other end of the stage, farthest from Blanche, emphasizing the separation that has occurred between the sisters.

This photo deserves commentary for another reason, however, since it captures an image of Blanche that represents what has happened to her in the play: she has been effectively silenced and removed from the group. Blanche's dialogue during the last scene has led progressively toward this final muteness, for her speeches are substantially shorter and less frequent here than elsewhere in the play. Her only extended dialogue in this scene is the speech in which she imagines her death at sea. Immediately afterwards, the Doctor and Nurse appear, and Blanche's disorientation about the turn of events dominates her remaining lines: "I—I—" and "I don't know you—I don't know you. I want to be—left alone—please!" (I, 415). Only in her famous exit line does she regain her composure in response to the Doctor's gentlemanly overture. "Whoever you are—I have always depended on the kindness of strangers," are her last words, and although this line has attained a stature awarded only to the most memorable lines in theater history, our last visual image of Blanche is her mute exit. In this final picture she is ignored by most of the other characters, who continue activities of life in the Quarter.

Blanche's journey toward this silent leave-taking at the corner of the stage is at the center of this drama, and the streetcar of the title foreshadows the mobility of her life. But we are not well prepared for her muteness, since her "garrulous" personality, to quote Ruby Cohn, has so dominated the stage (Cohn, *Dialogue* 97). Ironically, however, her excess of speech, her incessant storytelling, her insistence on holding the center of attention, underline her forced silence at the end of the play. Stanley's fury during the first poker scene arises in part from the chatter of the two sisters. Blanche asks if she can "kibitz," seeking to gain the players' attention; after she and Stella retire to the bedroom, Stanley attempts to silence their speech, shouting, "You hens cut out the conversation in there!" (I, 294). When the women turn on the radio, Stanley again shouts for silence: "Turn it off!" (I, 295). The noise continues as Mitch joins Blanche in the bedroom, and Blanche turns on the radio again: this time Stanley reacts with violence, storming into the bedroom, and tossing the radio out the window. This display not only demonstrates the force of Stanley's reaction to Blanche's earliest attempt to corner Mitch, it shows his response to unwanted noise: he disposes of it.

The next scene reinforces Stanley's convictions that Blanche talks too much, for he overhears one of her most extended speeches of the play; this lecture consists of a detailed condemnation of Stanley, in which she implores Stella not to "hang back with the brutes!" (I, 323). When Stella reminds Stanley in scene seven that "Blanche and I grew up under very different circumstances than you did," Stanley retorts, "So I been told. And told and told and told" (I, 358). During the birthday party scene, Stanley's second fit of destructive behavior is a reaction to the sisters' criticism of his habits. Apparently influenced by Blanche, Stella remarks that Stanley is "making a pig of himself," and tells him: "Go and wash up and then help me clear the table" (I, 371). Throwing a plate to the floor, he seizes Stella's arm: "Don't ever talk that way to me! 'Pig— Polack—disgusting—vulgar—greasy!'—them kind of words have been on your tongue and your sister's too much around here!" (I, 371). This speech emphasizes Stanley's resentment of the terms which Blanche (and now Stella) apply to him. In the first poker night scene, and in the one above, his physical violence is directed at Stella: in the former scene, he strikes her, and in the latter, he "seizes her arm" (I, 371).

Stanley reacts strongly to the character insults because he senses their truth; shortly after throwing the dishes, he admits to Stella to being "common as dirt." While he only begrudgingly admits to the truth about himself, however, he *insists* on knowing and exposing the truth about Blanche. Suspecting the counterfeit nature of her life's story, Stanley sets out to prove her a liar. Laura Morrow and Edward Morrow argue that "Stanley is passionately devoted to truth-seeing and truth-telling"; Blanche goes mad "when Stanley confronts her with the truth" (Morrow 59). Because she has embellished and glossed over the facts of her past, no one is compelled to believe her story about the rape; it is this story that precipitates her institutionalization.

In scene seven, when Stanley reveals his findings about Blanche to Stella, the latter denies the information about her sister's expulsion from Laurel. She calls Stanley's accusations "contemptible lies" and "pure invention." Having heard all of it, however, Stella does admit: "It's possible that some of the things he [the salesman] said are partly true" (I, 364). With her concession that Blanche's version of how and why she left Laurel may not be entirely accurate, Stella opens the floodgates for her final rejection of Blanche. Blanche tells one final story, that Stanley raped her on the night of the baby's birth; Stella rejects this account, having already acknowledged that Blanche has been fabricating other tales. The story of the rape, which Stella tells Eunice she cannot believe if she is to continue to live with Stanley, convinces Stella that she must participate in the act of Blanche's institutionalization. Although the audience/reader knows that this time Blanche does not lie, the conscience of the community, represented by Stella and Eunice, judges this story to be a falsehood. When the conscience of the community makes its verdict, then the confinement can take place without delay.

Blanche's insistence, therefore, on changing the past to agree with her image of herself as a proper gentlewoman, establishes the necessary precedent for Stella's denial of the rape. It is impossible to know what parts of Blanche's own character analysis are lies, and what stories result from self-delusion. When Mitch confronts her about her lies, she claims: "Never inside, I didn't lie in my heart" (I, 387). Although she insists that she has never been guilty of deliberate cruelty, she admits to Mitch that she prompted Allan's suicide by telling him, "You disgust me" (I, 355). Contradictory assertions seem to be symptomatic of her emotional disintegration; as all stability slips away from her, the statements she makes conflict with one another.

In *Streetcar*, Blanche's mental decline is apparent throughout the play; in the opening of scene ten, advanced deterioration is visible, only in part connected to her extreme drunkenness. As Stanley enters, she speaks "as if to a group of spectral admirers" (I, 391). Perhaps her confession to Mitch about her life in Laurel has propelled Blanche to the very brink of sanity; significantly, the former scene marks the first time that she tells the entire truth about her past. This combination of circumstances provides further evidence that telling the truth contributes to her downfall. Whatever the causes of this latest break with reality, she has succumbed to the illusion about Shep Huntleigh's rescue of her, and imagines that she is preparing to take a cruise. Although her loss of sanity seems evident, however, her departure to the state hospital is not made final until she exposes Stanley's violent act. Stanley has already proven to Stella and Mitch that Blanche lied about her life in Laurel; when the truth of the rape becomes an issue, they choose Stanley's story over that of Blanche.[1]

This predicament, the determination to choose one story over another, as well as the defensiveness of the one deemed mad because of the content of the account, is a source of tension in other plays as well. Although the process is reversed in *Suddenly Last Summer,* once again the sanity and the confinement of the presumed mad person depends on the story that is central to the play. An early draft, in which Catharine is named Valerie, focuses on her propensity to chatter, for she tells the sister who accompanies her from the institution: "I can't stop talking, I never could when I'm nervous."[2] Immediately after this, she informs the doctor that her nails have been cut to keep her from hurting herself during the convulsions that occur after shock treatment. The doctor then asks the sister, "Isn't she off shock now?" and Valerie replies: "You can ask me, I can answer. I'm off it now." This version emphasizes that the girl is ready and anxious to talk about her treatment, and to tell the story that has been her undoing; indeed, she will persist in telling her version of the truth no matter what: "They can't cut the true story out of my brain." Also: "I'm going to get the truth serum again I know. But it doesn't change the story." A longer speech about the story she is prepared to tell reveals her inner wrestling with the narrative of her cousin's fate:

I can't falsify it . . . It's no pleasure having to repeat the same story over and over, but even if I wished not to, even if I wished to falsify it, what could I say? . . . I just can't help repeating what actually did happen, it just—spills out!— each time!—the truth about what happened.[3]

Although Williams deletes these comments from the final version, he retains the concentration on truth; the word "truth" is repeated fifteen times, mostly by Catharine, and it is echoed by the doctor in the final line of the play: "I think we ought at least to consider the possibility that the girl's story could be true" (III, 423). Truth has "the last word." Its constant recurrence emphasizes its significance. Defining the truth may well determine Catharine's future.

In the earlier version, Valerie [Catharine] sums up the major conflict of the play when she tells the doctor, "I'm not mad. It's just that I witnessed something no one will believe and they'd rather think I'm mad than to believe it."[4] Her statement illustrates one of the most common determinations of madness in Williams's plays: whether an implausible story is accepted by the other characters. The predicament she describes could be that of either Blanche (although Blanche is more than a witness to the violent act in *Streetcar*), or Valerie [Catharine], for the latter assesses the truth as unbelievable; the only option for those who deny this truth is to proclaim the teller mad. In both plays, the madwoman insists on telling a story whose premise is unacceptable, thus resulting in that woman's expulsion from society. Allan Ingram in *The Madhouse of Language* writes: "one prime feature of the madman's discourse is obsession, the returning always to one subject of conversation" (38). Catharine's obsession with the story of Sebastian's death causes her to return to that subject incessantly; as Violet tells the Doctor, Catharine "babbles" it at every opportunity. Although we wonder about her sanity, we cannot deny her obsessive discourse.

In a review of the original production of *Suddenly,* Richard Watts describes the action as "in large part a drama of two speeches, the first by the mother of a dead poet, who is certain that a young woman has caused his death, and the other by the possibly insane girl, who gives her own version of what happened."[5] Like the rape in *Streetcar,* Sebastian's death is also a story of violence, as well as a narrative that maligns the character of the central male figure of the play. In *Suddenly,* however, Sebastian is dead, and cannot refute the tale's truth, as Stanley does. At *Suddenly*'s opening, Catharine is already confined for telling the story, and so the action contrasts with that of *Streetcar:* it moves toward the possible release of Catharine at the end of the play. The account that Catharine gives of Sebastian's death unequivocally provides the only reason for Catharine's confinement, although she does exhibit peculiar behavior: she causes a scene at a Mardi Gras ball, and she shows unusual distance from her own feelings by using the third-person in her diary. But her horrifying tale, with the aspersions it casts on Sebastian's character, sends her to the asylum and results in her receiving various treatments for memory suppression, attempts designed to prevent her from repeating her version of his murder.

The story prompts Violet Venable to seek the assistance of Doctor Cukrowicz, who performs lobotomies. If he can determine that Catharine has fabricated the story, he will perform the operation. In this play, two men represent the deciding consensus of the community: the doctor, and Catharine's brother, George. Unlike *Streetcar,* in *Suddenly* we do not know if the story is true, but we do get to hear Catharine tell it, and we also witness the reaction of her audience. In *Suddenly,* the story has strikingly different effects on the characters who hear it: Catharine's narrative sends Violet into a rage, demanding that the story be excised from her niece's brain; however, it seems to convince the doctor, who is at least ready to accept the possibility of its truth. George seems more convinced, even though his position throughout the play has been on the side of his aunt, since he wants the money from the inheritance.

These two plays make clear, in different ways, that the characters' ability to convince others of the truth of certain situations does not depend on whether these events actually occurred. Ultimately, this is because the line between truth and fiction often blurs. Tom Wingfield's description of the play he narrates gives a hint of this, when he claims it to be "truth in the pleasant guise of illusion," and Blanche provides another twist when she speaks of telling "what ought to be truth." Both *Streetcar* and *Suddenly* raise the possibility of confinement for a major character; what becomes clear, however, is that the confinement is decided in part because these women have forced others to consider how the truth might be determined.

One important distinction is noteworthy in a comparison of the storytelling aspects of the plays. We might contrast their dramatic progression by saying that Blanche moves toward madness, and Catharine moves away from it toward her possible release. Blanche's last long speech is not about the past, as the others have been, but about the future, a virtual prediction of her own death. In contrast, Catharine's longest speech occurs at the end of the play; she does not appear in the first scene, and in that scene Mrs. Venable controls the doctor's perceptions of Sebastian's character and life. Violet makes a reference to "talking the ears off a donkey," indicating an awareness of her verbosity. When the group has gathered to hear Catharine's version of the events in Cabeza de Lobo, Violet repeatedly interrupts Catharine's speeches, attempting to adjust or deny the girl's declarations. Finally the doctor halts the interruptions, and demands that Catharine be allowed to continue her narrative without interruption. Not only is the monologue the dramatic climax of the play, it allows the revelation of the story that has caused Catharine's confinement, a narrative that Violet seeks to silence. The release of this story to the ears of the family and the doctor (and the audience) thwarts Violet's effort to suppress it, and may lead to Catharine's release.

This situation contrasts with Blanche's circumstances in *Streetcar.* Although we see the rape, or at least its commencement, we do not hear Blanche tell of it later; all we know of Stella's reaction to it is that she rejects it, deciding to send her sister to an institution. Blanche's inability to find a sympathetic audience suggests that she is being sent away because she spoke of the rape, and broke the silence with her accusation against Stanley.

In both plays the confinement hinges on a story of an unmentionable act, a violation of an accepted societal taboo. Beyond the shock value of these acts, they have a common ground in violence and in their taboo elements. Their similarity implies that madness has connections to the unmentionable, that society seeks to suppress the language of madness because that language speaks of prohibited acts of sex and violence. Lucretia's confinement in *Portrait of a Madonna* can be seen in this light as well: although we are quite convinced that she fabricates her story about Richard's visits to "indulge his senses," the narrative has the taboo quality of the others, with its subject matter of rape and illegitimate conception. The madwomen in these three plays are put away in part because of the shocking stories they tell, which reveal unspeakable elements of human behavior. As Catharine claims of her narrative, "it's a true story of our time and the world we live in" (III, 382); this may be so, but the other characters refuse to admit it.

The situations that instigate the madwomen's confinement reveal a pattern that can be traced through some other Williams's plays. In *The Night of the Iguana,* Shannon tells his own version of the "forbidden act"; his act, like the others, is inextricably tied to his first confinement. Once more, a story of unacceptable behavior alarms the community, and they confine the person responsible for shocking them. Shannon's conduct with her young charge prompts Miss Fellowes to investigate his past. Shannon denies her accusations that he has been defrocked, even attempting to convince those around him of his current ministerial status. He insists to Hannah that he must wear his collar because, "I've been accused of being defrocked and of lying about it. I want to show the ladies that I'm still a clocked—*frocked!*—minister of the . . ." (IV, 300).

When questioned further on the subject by Hannah, he admits to being "inactive in the Church for all but one year since I was ordained a minister of the Church" (IV, 301). Her response: "Well, that's quite a sabbatical, Mr. Shannon," signifies that she will accept his version of his discharge. This tactic draws the story out of him, and he tells of his sexual transgression with a young Sunday-school teacher: "the natural, or unnatural, attraction of one . . . lunatic for . . . another" (IV, 303). His behavior elicits disapproval from the parishioners, to which he responds with a shocking sermon on "the *truth* about God!" [my emphasis] (IV, 304). Despite a difference in magnitude, perhaps, Shannon's story shares qualities with the others in Williams's plays. Most important for this analysis, Shannon's attempt to warn his parishioners results in his confinement: "Well, I wasn't defrocked. I was just locked out of the church in Pleasant Valley, Virginia, and put in a nice little private asylum to recuperate from a complete nervous breakdown as they preferred to regard it" (IV, 304).

Although Shannon's affair with the young woman earns their "smug, disapproving, accusing faces," his attempts to enlighten them about the Western concept of God as a "senile delinquent," an "angry, petulant old man," brings about his institutionalization.

As these plays illustrate, honest expression threatens those who reveal what they consider the truth, when that expression affronts the members of society who are considered normal. Only Lucretia's story about Richard is quite clearly false; what it explains about her lonely, isolated life, however, is undeniably revealing. What the reception of these narratives explains about the fear and narrowness of the communities who reject the tellers is as crucial to our understanding of the plays as our attempt to analyze the emotional instability of the characters deemed mad. Viewed this way, madness becomes the social category created for dealing with these rebels; the confinement which results from this labeling provides a method for insuring their silence. The play's form, however, contradicts this silence: in most cases, the audience witnesses the release of the truth. The community of the play denies the story, but from our vantage point outside the action, we see its effect on the society of the drama. Although the characters deemed mad speak of their weaknesses, their frailties, they prove stronger than their "normal" counterparts, for they willingly face the unpalatable. *Iguana* stands apart from the other plays, for in Hannah Jelkes, Shannon finds a sympathetic audience who does not spurn his story.

The Two-Character Play provides another example of the taboo narrative, for Felice and Clare of the play-within-the-play have a sordid tale of their own to tell, or to hide. Their father's murder/suicide of his wife and himself constitutes their story of family horror; like the other characters I have discussed, they cannot help but be obsessed by the incident, even though they are aware of its part in isolating them from the community of New Bethesda. Clare insists on mentioning the "terrible accident" when she calls the Reverend Wiley, and Felice accuses her of "babbling" to him. They cannot find a way to reconcile the story with their relationship in the world, specifically to the insurance company that will not honor their father's insurance policy.

With this dilemma, *The Two-Character Play* highlights another issue of language and madness: the brother and sister struggle constantly with certain kinds of language. When they discuss the insurance policy that has been forfeited because their father killed his wife, then himself, Clare cannot find the correct language, the official language to describe the rejection of their claim. The Acme Insurance Company has notified them by mail about the denial:

> Clare: —what's the word? Confiscated?
> Felice: Forfeited.
> Clare: Yes, the payment of the insurance policy is forfeited in the—what is the word?
> Felice: Event.
> Clare : Yes, in the event of a man—[*She stops, pressing her fist to her mouth.*] (V, 343)

Clare lacks the proper official language of the insurance company, the bureaucratic language with which they deny payment. Beyond that, she finds it impossible to tell the horrible story with which she and her brother are obsessed.

Williams states in the author's notes of the 1970 manuscript version: "'Grossman's Market' (and its proprietor) and 'The Acme Insurance Company' represent formidable and impersonal forces in the lives of the two characters."[6] Williams also points out in his notes that the "Acme" responds to a twelve-page written and rewritten letter of appeal with only three typewritten sentences. The "Acme" speaks with the voice of authority, the voice of reason: it follows strict guidelines about paying claims. When Felice and Clare speak of the insurance company's response, Felice argues: "[T]here are situations in which legal technicalities have to be, to be—disregarded in the interests of human, human—"; however, Clare rightly answers him, "[Y]ou under-esteem the, the—power of a company called *The Acme*."[7] Clare notes the disparity between the twelve-page appeal and the three sentence response, which indicates that the emotional language of the disturbed and isolated survivors, holds no weight for the businesslike approach of the company.

Felice and Clare speak of lying to the insurance company, and likewise, about lying to Mr. Grossman about whether they will be paid the money from Acme. Once more we see that the truth becomes a barometer of insanity; if Felice and Clare relate the true circumstances of their parents' death, the insurance company can label the family disturbed and be rid of them with a terse, official note. Its opinion will then influence other institutions, such as Grossman's market, spreading outward to the members of the community. If the surviving siblings can convince "Acme" of a more acceptable version of the circumstances that justify the claim, they might be entitled to some monetary compensation that would allow them once more to be paying customers at the market. Like the characters of the other plays, however, Felice and Clare cannot alter their story in order to accommodate the norms of the community.

This is just one case of the brother and sister's failure to use language to their advantage. Felice and Clare are constantly stymied by the absence of the language that they need to convince others to help them. When they receive the telegram from their theater company, accusing them of being insane, they cannot respond to these accusations, because the company chooses a one-sided method of communication to state their grievances. During the play-within-the-play, the other Felice and Clare often argue about the effects that their cries for help may have on those they ask. When the representatives from "Citizens Relief" come calling, Felice and Clare cannot face them, so they do not answer the door. When they speak afterward of the possibility of asking the group for help, they are hesitant because of what they might have to say to them:

> Clare: Oh, but all the questions we'd have to—
> Felice: Answer.
> Clare: Yes, there'd be interviews and questionnaires to fill out and—
> Felice: Organizations are such—
> Clare: *Cold!*
> Felice: Yes, impersonal things. (V, 333)

They are afraid of what they might have to tell the group in order to receive help, and as in the case of the insurance company, they know enough not to expect human warmth from an organization. They cannot make their needs known to anyone lacking compassion for their troubled and battered psyches.

Clare suspects that this kind of compassion may be available from the Reverend Wiley, although his name alerts us that this is rather doubtful. Sy Kahn notes the comparison between the names of the stage manager (Fox) and the minister, suggesting that both might be "wily foxes" (50). Clare's call to the minister is the first and only time the brother or sister make outside contact with anyone, although they speak of doing so throughout the inner play. Felice does not want Clare to call the Reverend, for when she tells the operator to put her through to him, "Felice tries to wrest the phone from her grasp, and for a moment they struggle for it"(V, 337). Clare insists that Felice let her talk: "You'll have to let me go on or he'll think I'm—" (V, 337). Clare speaks to the Reverend about the charges against her father, and the subsequent results of these charges on the lives of his children. Insisting on the false nature of these accusations, she speaks of their struggles to exist "surrounded by so much suspicion and malice" (V, 337). Felice grabs the phone from her, makes an excuse of illness to Wiley, and hangs up. He complains to Clare that "our one chance is privacy and you babble away to a man who'll think it his Christian duty to have us *confined* in—" (V, 338). Clearly, Felice believes that any talking they might do will only decrease their chances of remaining free; communication with others will not help them, but will contribute to their doom.

After Felice and Clare have abandoned hope of taking a trip to Grossman's market, not only because they cannot go out, but because they cannot face speaking to Grossman about their need for more credit, they consider asking for assistance from "Citizens' Relief." The name suggests the impossibility of this idea, for they are no longer citizens. They do not belong to the community, but are set apart from them, and can expect no aid; they cannot even request it. If they could, they might still be part of the community. Once they decide to attempt such a plea, their phone is dead. Felice suggests that Clare go next door and ask to use the neighbors' phone, and tells Clare to call out to the neighbor woman, who is in the yard. Clare attempts to address her, but cannot speak loudly enough to be heard. Her "outcry" does not go out, and when Felice tells her: "Not loud enough, call louder," she turns from the window. She sums up the impossibility of their situation: "Did you really imagine that I could call and beg for Citizens' Relief in front of those malicious people next door, on their phone, in their presence?" (V, 355).

Although Felice and Clare have lost the ability to communicate with others, they *can* speak to each other. The whole play consists of the communication between these deranged characters. By peopling this play with only two characters, whose sanity is questionable, Williams concentrates on creating a private language between people who need not worry about outside interference. In this play, Williams employs his common tactic of frequent dashes, marking incomplete sentences; here it does not signify a difficulty of communication, but the opposite, since Felice and Clare are close enough to interpret one another's unspoken words. An element of theatrical self-consciousness complicates this impression; when Felice and Clare act out the inner play, they are aware of each other's words because of the script they have memorized. The script is in a state of flux, however, because of Clare's insistence on improvisation, and even when they "come out" of the play, they anticipate each other's words.

The unfinished sentences and emphasis on the unspoken word appear in another play of this period, *In the Bar of a Tokyo Hotel*. By comparing the two, we see the way that Williams has used this technique with effectiveness in *The Two-Character Play,* while in the other work the same half-sentence construction lends only incoherence to the text.[8] Throughout *In the Bar of a Tokyo Hotel,* everyone speaks in incomplete sentences, although only Mark, the ravaged artist, appears to suffer from psychological problems. The reader or audience is puzzled, then, about why the characters stop mid-sentence or why another character jumps in to finish another's thoughts. In both plays, the device seems to indicate the verbal incapacity of the characters, as well as the inadequacy of language to express their state of emotional turmoil. Williams achieves more consistency, as well as more significance, when he uses this verbal technique in *The Two-Character Play.* When Felice and Clare cut short their sentences, they exhibit their fears of the things they dare not speak; they demonstrate their frozen psychological state; they convey the unspeakable terror of their situation. Likewise, when they help each other finish sentences, they indicate their interwoven lives and personalities, and their limited ability to aid each other in communication. Although they have been cut off from the world, both in the outer play and the inner one, communication may be difficult, but it is still possible between them.

Discussion of this linguistic feature of *The Two-Character Play* suggests that consideration of other features of language might be appropriate to an analysis of madness in the texts of this study. Allan Ingram writes on the writing and reading of madness in the eighteenth century:

We should not deny the existence of madness as something that is also beyond the framework of a linguistic construct. The experience of pain and of mental suffering must always proceed in a region that is remote from language, even if the sufferer attempts to retrieve that experience through the medium of language. (8)

In looking at Williams's plays, then, we might consider how the playwright overcomes the obstacle of language in relation to madness: can madness be expressed through a language governed by principles of reason? Is it possible for the mad to reach across the division that separates them from the sane and express the experience of madness? What's more, can the characters of a drama present themselves as mad, and still speak in a language comprehensible to the audience? Perhaps Williams's isolation of Felice and Clare in *The Two-Character Play* represents an attempt to set their language apart: as long as no other characters interact with the deranged brother and sister, their communication exists apart from the world. Although Felice and Clare show confusion and fear in their speeches, we do not hear lunatic ravings. This holds true for all the mad characters of Williams's plays, leading to the conclusion that Williams by and large does not succeed in dramatizing madness at the level of language use.

This being said, however, we may still examine the linguistic features that the playwright employs to invoke the nervousness and levels of delusion that we recognize as his attempts to have his characters vocalize their emotional instability. Williams's early characters often speak in an artificial manner: Alma Winemiller is accused by others as being affected and self-consciously pretentious in her speech. Blanche also uses the flowery language of a past age, in part an attribute of these women's southern heritage. Both Alma and Blanche, however, are noted for their nervous, hysterical characters; their tendency towards hyperbole is intertwined with southern gentility and emotional extremity. Thus, in *Eccentricities of a Nightingale,* Alma's father tells her: "The thing for you to give up is your affectations, Alma . . . that make you seem— well—slightly *peculiar* to people! . . . You, you, you—*gild the lily! . . .* you—stammer, you—laugh hysterically and clutch at your throat!" (II, 32). Exaggeration is a trait of eccentricity, and Alma's strangeness cannot be separated from her verbal mannerisms.

Blanche also exaggerates, but while her verbal extravagance is, like Alma's, a plea for attention, her extreme comments about herself tragically foreshadow her fate. She tells Stella: "I was on the verge of—lunacy, almost!"; "Daylight never exposed so total a ruin!"; "I want to be *near* you, got to be *with* somebody, I *can't* be *alone!*" (I, 254, 257). However, Blanche's ability to describe her mental condition deteriorates at the play's ending, when, mute and lost in illusion, she is led off by the Doctor.

The faltering quality of the dialogue is another feature distinctive of Williams. Rarely has a playwright employed more dashes or ellipses to demonstrate nervousness, indecision, and hesitation. These traits are attributable to the characters who find themselves at the end of their rope, and are confused or lost about where or how to proceed. The verbal hesitations signify the inner hesitation, and convey to the audience the loss of purpose or direction that marks the wandering mind. Williams's use of this kind of verbal reluctance represents his version of loss of expression. The mad characters in Williams's plays are rarely silent, as Blanche is at the conclusion of *Streetcar*; on the contrary, they have ways of illustrating their mental incapacities.

Clothes for a Summer Hotel marks both similarities and differences with the earlier plays about madness. In this late play, Williams writes of the Zelda Fitzgerald who has been institutionalized; yet, of all the characters in the play, she is the most perceptive and the most vocal about human failings and the limitations of relationships. Scott, the "sane" partner in their marriage, comes to the hospital "dressed as if about to check in at a summer hotel" (*Clothes* 9). He becomes excited and disturbed when unrecognized, then presumed drunk, by Dr. Zeller; Scott suffers further indignities in Act two, when he has another conversation with the doctor, the latter insisting on the superiority of Zelda's novel: "Zelda has sometimes struck a sort of fire in her work that—I'm sorry to say this to you, but I never quite found anything in yours, even yours, that was—equal to it" (55). Scott, the successful writer, master of language, does not measure up to his wife's abilities to lure this reader.

In the couple's verbal matches, Zelda more often emerges superior as well as more honest. She speaks truthfully of her estrangement from Scott, while he "draws back wounded" when she pointedly describes their embrace as a "meaninglessly conventional—gesture" (10). She acknowledges that her continued confinement depends on society's labeling of her: "I only come back here when I know I'm too much for Mother and the conventions of Montgomery, Alabama. I am pointed out on the street as a lunatic now" (11). Voicing her belief that she did not provide the best atmosphere for Scott's work, she confesses to him that he "needed a better influence, someone much more stable as a companion on the—roller-coaster ride which collapsed at the peak" (15). In all these statements about her illness and the collapse of their marriage, Zelda speaks with perceptive self-knowledge and brutal honesty. Near the close of the first scene, Williams's stage directions indicate what we have come to suspect: according to him, madness is a social category, highly ambiguous and questionable. The playwright does so with a slight, almost imperceptible gesture, which gains significance upon close examination of Zelda's character. When Zelda speaks of life in the asylum, Williams notes that "Zelda must somehow suggest the desperate longing of the 'insane' to communicate something of their private world to those from whom they're secluded" (26). By placing quotation marks around the word "insane," Williams calls into question the label he has used to define his most memorable characters. This note likewise highlights the aspect of communication that is so crucial to the understanding of the verbal struggles of those who are called mad. Finally, Williams insists that Zelda's words in this section are not crucial, "mostly blown away by the wind," but her eyes and her gestures "must win the audience to her inescapably from this point in the play" (26). As with Blanche's mute exit, when her image replaces her verbal power to convince us, Zelda's presence must argue her position.

While Zelda's words are swallowed by the wind here, however, she remains the most vocal character in the play, explaining her life and her destiny. Her eloquence in the final scene, where she speaks of mad-

ness, art, life, and death, reveals her superior vision, having been "puri-
fied by madness and by fire" (9). Zelda places herself in the tradition of
the mad seer, telling Scott of her death by fire, aware of this because
"the demented often have the gift of Cassandra, the gift of—Premo-
nition!" (15). Her perceptive outlook on the past and the future reveals
her more capable than Scott of acknowledging the truth about their marriage and his career.

Finally, the play resembles the others in this discussion, with its use
of the sexual transgression as secret and truth revealed. Zelda's affair
with Edouard, a French aviator, dominates the action of the two middle
scenes, with the intern from the asylum doubling as Edouard; this tactic
blurs the boundaries of past and present. Although Scott knows of the
affair, Edouard worries about her husband's reaction; as the intern, he
speaks of Scott: "*Pauvre homme.* I was always concerned. Wondered
what effect the indiscretion—" (25). The affair lacks the violence, the
horror of narratives from the other plays, but it has its part in Zelda's
institutionalization. She claims her infidelity sets off her madness, for the
end of the affair prompts her to attempt suicide; she tells Scott that when
Edouard rejected her, "I think my heart died and I—went—mad" (59).
Given Zelda's clear-headed responses to all that happens around her, her
madness is questionable. Perhaps, however, this is as it should be: her
institutionalization provides the consummate example of the fate of the
sensitive individual who cannot find a suitable outlet for her passions.
Although confined, she remains cognizant of her situation; like Catharine
Holly, she cannot keep from protesting the truth of her experience.

In creating characters who persist, despite great difficulty, in proclaiming "true stories of our time and the world we live in," Williams
demonstrates his conviction that American society seeks to silence those
who shock or outrage with stories of the unmentionable. By establishing
these narratives as intrinsic parts of the action, by hanging the fate of the
characters on the telling of these tales, the playwright creates situations
in which those who bear witness to the atrocities of human action find
their sanity questioned, their words muted. Like the fools in Shakespeare's plays, these characters and their truths are disregarded or disbe-
lieved. Unlike Shakespeare, however, where the fools' warnings predict
the downfall of the characters who ignore them, Williams's "fools" and
their babbling affect their own destiny, usually adversely.

4

Deranged Artists: Creativity and Madness

The lunatick, the lover and the poet
Are of imagination all compact.
—*A Midsummer Night's Dream*

Writers are often quite naturally preoccupied with the creative process, and Tennessee Williams was no exception: he demonstrated his interest in the artist's role in society by addressing the issue in his plays. George Niesen writes that although not all of Tennessee Williams's plays feature an artist, "most of the plays include someone in the cast with the qualities—if not the title—of an artist. In each case the figure is sensitive, creative, and, paradoxically, destructive" (463). While Niesen's study broadens the definition of the artist figure to include anyone who demonstrates a proclivity to art, my discussion will be limited to those who have created works of art, especially literary ones. Niesen argues in his essay that the artists in Williams's early plays die because of their sensitivity, and in the later plays, these artists are "angels of death," for they bring about the death of others (463). While Niesen's essay is the most detailed about the artist figure in Williams's plays, he does not examine the link between artistry and madness.

Although the artist's relationship to madness is a major concern in a number of Williams's plays, critical attention has been slight in this area. The neglect of the topic may be due to the tendency of Williams's critics to treat madness as a peripheral issue in his plays. Another reason may be the ambiguity of Williams's treatment of madness and creativity: the need to create art can be the source of both mental anguish and salvation. While Williams acknowledges the stereotype of mad artist as pervasive in Western literature, at other times he suggests that artistic creation may provide a means of keeping madness at bay. After a survey of theories on creativity and madness, an exploration of the representative plays will clarify the position Williams's dramas endorse.

The theoretical information available on the connection between madness and artistic creativity is abundant, and the discussion of their relationship spans centuries. In a chapter on "Madness and Genius" in his book *The Social History of Madness,* Roy Porter contrasts the views of Plato and Aristotle on the relationship of madness and art; although both have different views on the source of the creative spirit, they align that creative spirit with madness (60-61). Porter claims that Plato saw genius sparked by a "mystical heaven-sent spirit or *furor,* through which a select few could be 'inspired'"; for Aristotle, "'melancholy' was both a disposition and, almost, a disease . . . In a few, that moody, broody, pensive streak proved highly creative in images and ideas; it was the humor of genius" (60-61). In neither case do we have the exact corollary to our modern understanding of madness: in the first case Plato assigns inspiration to a divine source, and in the second, Aristotle's position, Porter rightly notes, lies within the "tradition of classical medical thinking about man associated with his name" (61).

Porter briefly chronicles the pendulum swing of attitudes toward madness and creativity in Western literature, claiming that "it is with Romanticism, of course, that the indissoluble link between madness and artistic genius comes into its own as an autobiographical experience, even as the armorial bearings of talent" (63). This position compares more closely to the view of insanity and madness which has directed the dialogue in our time. Two aspects of this theory have survived to the present: "that madness (or, more generally, great torment) is the anvil of noble art," and "the Promethean one that madness is the price to be paid for creation" (63).

Porter does not speak specifically about the modern age and its attitudes, but studies of the artist in contemporary society suggest that this Romantic notion has remained with us. In *Madness and Modernism,* Louis A. Sass speaks of the basic assumption that madness is irrationality: "a condition involving decline or even disappearance of the role of rational factors in the organization of human conduct and experience." Sass sees this definition of madness as the absence of rationality, "the core idea that, in various forms but with few true exceptions, has echoed down through the ages." Along with this conception, however, comes the vision of the mad person as "a prophet in the grip of demonic forces . . . associated with insight and vitality but also with blindness, disease, and death" (1).

Sass's purpose is not to argue for one or the other but rather to explore particular aspects of schizophrenia (on which he chooses to focus) by comparing them to various tenets of modernist art. In fact, Sass specifically states in his introduction that he does not "wish to glorify schizophrenic forms of madness—to argue, for example, that they are especially conducive to artistic creativity" (9). He mentions Tennessee Williams's *Suddenly Last Summer* and a reference to madness in the film version of the play; having mentioned other writers, Sass lumps them together and claims that their literary conceptions of madness have no experiential base, for most of these writers "have had little or no experience with the realities of chronic insanity" (4). About Tennessee Williams, he could not be more wrong.

A recent work by Albert Rothenberg specifically dealing with creativity and madness disputes the stereotype of genius arising out of lunacy. Using as evidence the same quotation from *A Midsummer's Night Dream* with which I began this chapter, he claims: "The idea of mad genius has long been popularly accepted in both our culture and our literature" (6). He claims that deviant behavior, "whether in the form of eccentricity or worse, is not only associated with persons of genius or high-level creativity, but it is frequently expected of them" (149). Rothenberg assigns these ideas to myth, arguing that "key aspects of creative thinking have nothing really to do with psychosis" (12). The book studies successful creative thinkers (his emphasis is primarily artistic, but he also includes scientific creativity in his assertions) and schizophrenics; the author maintains that although we link madness and creativity because creative thinking is characterized by its ability to look beyond the rational for new insights, and we associate madness with thinking beyond the rational, actually the key components of creative thinking are rational.

Rothenberg identifies an important creative cognitive sequence as the "janusian process," named after Janus, the Roman god of doorways whose two faces look in opposite directions at the same time. He then argues: "Contrary to the romantic notion that creativity grows largely out of inspiration, the thinking of dreams, or some unconscious source . . . the janusian process—a major element of the creative process—[is] a conscious, rational process" (15). In this process, "multiple opposites or antitheses are conceived simultaneously, either as existing side by side or as equally operative, valid, or true" (15). Rothenberg does not believe this process is illogical or irrational but rather a conscious formulation of the "simultaneous operation of antithetical elements or factors"; the artist "develops those formulations into integrated entities and creations" (15). When Rothenberg conducted a study comparing the thought processes of Nobel laureates, undergraduates from Yale, and psychiatric patients, he concluded that the first two groups showed tendencies to use the janusian type of thinking, but the psychiatric patients did not (23).

Another component of his research that helped him to formulate these distinctions between the schizophrenic and the creative personality concerns a study of psychiatric patients in a hospital setting who attended class and were encouraged to write poetry. While some of

Rothenberg's assessments of the poetry they produced are not relevant to my topic, one of his comments is pertinent to Tennessee Williams's own work habits. While commenting on the uneven quality of the poetry these patients produced, and explaining how the psychiatrists/teachers offered feedback to the students/patients on their work, Rothenberg adamantly insists that after exciting interest in improving the poem, "a major hurdle appears . . . schizophrenic patients won't revise" (63). If he is correct in this assertion, then the schizophrenic artistic experience is far removed from the creative process that Williams himself engaged in: Williams revised continuously, often working for years on the same material in different forms. One play highlighted in this chapter, *The Two-Character Play,* constitutes a prime example of this, for the work exists in a number of versions, and in one version is retitled *Out Cry.* My interest does not lie, of course, in demonstrating the sanity of Williams the playwright, but this theory of Rothenberg's about the lack of revision among patients does seem to indicate that, however much Williams questioned his own sanity, in his artistic habits he did not fit with Rothenberg's assessments of the schizophrenics studied.

One other subject Rothenberg explores is directly relevant to the experience of Williams the playwright, and should be touched on, since Rothenberg mentions Williams a number of times in his chapter on homosexuality. Although Rothenberg admits that he does not intend to characterize homosexuality as madness, he includes homosexuality in his study, for he defines madness in the broadest sense: "all the designations of aberration, deviance, and malfunction that Western civilization has managed to connect to its hallowed faculties of genius and creativity" (13). He considers homosexuality to be one of many life situations that is responsible for conflict, and argues that this kind of conflict often translates into artistic experience. This theory coincides with Williams's contention that what he wrote came out of the experiences of his life, and that he tried to tell the truth about the world as he saw it. But perhaps his fears and preoccupation with madness are closer to the center of his work than his anxieties or conflicts about homosexuality. Both subjects appear in his work, but my discussion focuses on madness, and I do not include homosexuality as a form of "aberration."

The theoretical discussions outlined above provide some indication about how a close study of madness and the artist might illuminate Williams's work. Porter's summation of popular Romantic attitudes about madness certainly applies to the themes of Williams's plays, for the notion that art emerges from great torment (often related to madness), and that creativity emerges at the price of madness, figures in Williams's view of suffering as a great teacher. Edmund Wilson makes this point in his discussion of Sophocles' *Philoctetes* in *The Wound and the Bow,* for he maintains that it would occur to the modern reader that "genius and disease, like strength and mutilation, may be inextricably bound up together" (289). In Williams's plays, the characters who suffer the most have the deepest insights, and are undoubtably the emotional center of the plays. Madness as a cost of artistic creation is a subject touched on in a number of Williams's dramas, and is a central focus of *The Two-Character Play.* Sharing equal standing with this idea, how-ever, is the suggestion that the artist escapes madness because of the cre-ative spirit that keeps him focused on work, and out of the asylum (although sometimes by a narrow margin).

Personal and autobiographical factors enter into this last theory, for Williams insisted often that his writing helped keep him out of the asy-lums where his sister Rose spent most of her life.[1] In a study of literature that deals with psychiatric case studies, Jeffrey Berman claims that psy-chological illness "may promote scientific and artistic creativity by encouraging adaptive and integrative solutions to inner conflict" (27). Continuing along this line of thought, Berman might be describing Williams when he asserts that writers have "many reasons to write about mental breakdown, including the desire to exorcise old demons and ward off new ones" (27). But Williams's plays must also be examined as more than acts of personal therapy for the writer, and this chapter will be an attempt to formulate a statement about how madness relates to a variety of artist figures in his plays.

My discussion begins with one of Williams's most enduring and popular plays, which introduces the playwright's alter ego, the poet Tom Wingfield. *The Glass Menagerie* was Williams's first successful play, opening in New York in 1945; *Menagerie* is considered a thinly dis-guised version of Williams's own family life in St. Louis. One of the complications that arises immediately in discussing the autobiographical origins of the play comes with determining how much Laura resembles Williams's sister Rose. Laura is physically crippled, shy, and withdrawn; she hides in the St. Louis apartment, content to play with her glass fig-ures and listen to the victrola. Williams's sister, although not physically disabled, was emotionally unstable. The question is whether we can assume Rose's problems to be Laura's problems—is Laura mentally ill? If so, does Tom's escape from the family contribute to Laura's final col-lapse; furthermore, does Tom's own sanity make this escape necessary?

Some critics conclude that Laura is mentally ill. Thomas L. King, for example, sets up the connection between the artist and the disturbed relative in his essay on *The Glass Menagerie.* King argues that scene three of the play "begins with Tom writing, Tom the artist, and in it we see how the artistic sensibility turns a painful situation into 'art' by using distance" (87). King continues by contrasting Tom and Laura, calling her a "severely disturbed woman," whereas Tom is not similarly disturbed because he makes art (87).

King elaborates on the differences between Tom and Laura by comparing them to real-life relatives James Joyce and his daughter, Lucia, who was treated by Jung for severe mental problems. Jung wrote about the situation, comparing the father and daughter, maintaining that Joyce had a schizophrenic style, but he willed it and developed it consciously, which gave him control over his psychosis; Lucia, meanwhile "'was not a genius like her father, but merely a victim of her disease'" (87). In comparing these couples, King argues: "Jung's theory is a psychoanalyst's perception of the problem of artist and non-artist which is much the same as the problem of Tom and Laura" (87). His suggestion is, then, that the brother and sister in the play are both susceptible to mental illness, by virtue of heredity and family experience, but Tom escapes psychosis because he finds an outlet for his anxieties.

King's argument suggests a number of issues that are central to the study of the artist in Williams's plays, but before I consider the validity of the contrast King draws between the artist and the mad person who does not write, I need to consider further the critics' position on Laura's sanity. C. W. E. Bigsby also connects Laura with Rose, but he does not make explicit what he thinks Laura's fate might be. He admits that Laura and Amanda suffer from Tom's need to escape, stating that "the world closes in on Amanda and Laura as Tom offers them up as sacrifices to his art and his freedom" (Bigsby 2: 40). Bigsby goes on to claim:

Laura is a loving portrait of Williams' own sister locked up in her own inner world, her lobotomy trapping her in a permanent adolescence. It is a withdrawal from sociality for which Williams offers a gentler image, in terms of Laura's limp, an imperfection less intrusive, less totally disabling, but the play is a homage to her. (48)

Bigsby's comments are typical of the critics' logic that if *Menagerie* is autobiographical, and Laura is Rose, then Laura is disturbed mentally to the extent of withdrawing completely from life. Joseph K. Davis, in an essay about the play, says Laura "withdraws into the world of her glass animals, and so flees into a no-time of approaching mental collapse" (194). Rather than similarly claiming that Laura and Rose are alike in their mental conditions, I would argue that we cannot know exactly what will happen to Laura when Tom leaves the family at the end of the play, but that the play provides enough clues to indicate that

Laura's mental stability is as fragile as her glass figures, and that her inability to provide for herself makes her a likely candidate for an institution.

Laura's fear of others and inability to pursue either a career or a suitable marriage partner indicate that she may indeed fulfill the prophecy her mother predicts for her after the "fiasco" at Rubicam's Business College. Amanda suggests that Laura's insistence on staying home might well result in a life of dependence, and claims to have seen evidence of this kind of life, the life of "barely tolerated spinsters . . . stuck away in some little mousetrap of a room . . . little birdlike women without any nest" (I, 156).

As we saw in both *Streetcar* and *Portrait of a Madonna,* Williams believes that a woman without economic means may end up at the state asylum. Laura's nearly pathological shyness and inability to cope with life's pressures predispose her to such a fate. Near the end of the play, right after Jim tells Laura that he cannot call on her because of his tie to Betty, the scenic directions explain that the "holy candles in the altar of Laura's face have been snuffed out" (I, 230). The next screen legend to appear, just as Amanda enters the room, explains, "Things have a way of turning out so badly," and Amanda inadvertently underscores this with her lemonade song: "Good enough for any old maid" (I, 231). Thus, when Tom instructs Laura to blow out her candles at the close of the play, Jim's rejection, things turning out so badly, and Amanda's song about an old maid all conspire to suggest what Laura's future holds for her. Once Jim leaves, Amanda's first words reiterate the outcome, both of the evening with Jim, and probably, life, by repeating the words of the legend: "Things have a way of turning out so badly" (I, 234).

Amanda's speech in scene two follows Laura's description of the days that she spent while pretending to be attending the business school; these days were filled with trips to the zoo, and to the Jewel Box, "that big glass house where they raise the tropical flowers" (I, 155). Laura is associated with these locations and thus with enclosed spaces, the zoo complete with bars, and the Jewel Box, a place for observation of rare objects. Throughout the play, Laura is linked with her glass menagerie, so the zoo becomes a pertinent symbol for her possible fate.[2] These images cannot prove that Laura ends up in an asylum, but they do compare her to the confined animals, and Amanda's speech about the trapped life of a spinster confirms that comparison. However, at this point in the play, Laura's fate is not yet determined, and Amanda's desperate attempts to provide security for her daughter shift focus from pursuing a career to obtaining a husband, Laura's only other option.

This consideration of Laura's impossible future without a career or a marriage connects Laura to the women discussed in chapter 3, for without an income or the protection of family members, she becomes vulnerable to institutionalization, and thus her encounter with Jim becomes all the more poignant. We cannot speculate whether Jim might have saved Laura from the loneliness of her life in the apartment if he were not already engaged, but we are sure that this is the only chance Laura has for escape. Once Tom leaves, no more gentleman callers will appear, for Laura is too withdrawn and isolated to attract them herself.

When Amanda helps Laura to dress before Jim's arrival, and the stage directions indicate that a "fragile, unearthly prettiness has come out in Laura" (I, 191), Amanda undercuts the hope in this transformation by exclaiming to her daughter that this is "the prettiest you will ever be!" (I, 192). This remark differs from Amanda's other assessments of Laura, for she is more inclined to overrate her daughter. In the opening scene: "I want you to stay fresh and pretty—for gentleman callers!" even though none are expected (I, 147). When Tom calls her "different," Amanda replies: "I think the difference is all to her advantage" (I, 187). In the moments before Laura's touching encounter with her one and only gentleman caller, however, Amanda indicates that Laura's attractiveness is momentary.

We might use Amanda as an example of what happens to Laura, for although readers of the play do not question Amanda's sanity, and Williams characterizes her as someone with "endurance," he also claims that "having failed to establish contact with reality," Amanda "continues to live vitally in her illusions" (I, 129). Amanda's focus on her past as a young debutante in Mississippi closely allies her with such madwomen as Blanche and Lucretia, and her appearance in her cotillion dress when Jim arrives provides evidence that she lacks sense and acts inappropriately. In her strength and ability to endure, however, she resembles Williams's later characters, who despite their eccentricities and illusions, do not succumb to madness but continue to struggle in the world. Laura lacks Amanda's determination, however, and her endurance is questionable.

Although Amanda concerns herself with economic realities, and is careful to make "plans and provisions," she depends on Tom for economic survival as much as Laura does, and shows scant evidence that she could support herself. She did have a job demonstrating brassieres when Laura first started business college, but she no longer has that job, and we don't know why. In a letter to Audrey Wood, written on Metro-Goldwyn stationery, Williams outlines the scenes of the play for her. In this version, still entitled *The Gentleman Caller,* Williams notes in the outline of scene two that when Amanda comes home and confronts Laura about business college, "Amanda has been working as a model for matron's dresses at down-town dept. store and has just lost the job because of faded appearance."[3] She attempts to sell magazine subscriptions by phone, but with little apparent success. We hear two separate calls: the first woman hangs up on her, and the second pitch ends before we know what response she will get. From her nonstop chatter on both calls, we surmise that she is a nuisance to these women, and that her sales career would not sustain her in the absence of Tom's salary. Comparing Amanda with Laura, then, it seems safe to assume that Laura would be even less effective at supporting herself.

When Tom directs Laura to blow out her candles at the close of the play, it is more than a stage direction to secure lights out; the blackout occurs in Laura's briefly lit life as well. Since she cannot escape the apartment and her limited life there, by either a career or a husband, and since Tom, the breadwinner, has left the family, Laura's existence is tenuous. Her emotional stability is questionable, and she loses her brother's financial and emotional support. What is left to be considered is whether Laura's emotional instability and Tom's artistic talents stem from a single source, and whether Tom sacrifices her future to ensure his as an artist.

In *Creative Malady,* George Pickering speculates whether or not "illness, and particularly psychological illness, may sometimes be an aid to creative work" (17). Looking at the lives of a selection of creative and influential people, including Darwin and Freud, Pickering concludes that passion is the "chief characteristic . . . which relates the psychoneuroses of the characters here described and the creative work which brought them fame. In brief, a psychoneurosis represents passion thwarted, a great creative work, passion fulfilled" (309). Do Tom and Laura prove Pickering's theory?

Scene one is the only scene in the play in which Amanda, Laura, and Tom interact as a family. After Tom's opening monologue as narrator, he joins his sister and his mother at the dinner table. Although the togetherness of the meal is soon cut short by Tom's abrupt departure from the table, and he finishes out the scene standing by the portieres, the stage directions inform us that Amanda continues to address him "as though he were seated in the vacant chair at the table though he remains by the portieres" (I, 148). More importantly, though, the characters have their only three-way conversation of the play, on a well-rehearsed subject, Amanda's life in Blue Mountain. In this scene, then, Tom and Laura are brother and sister, participating in a familiar family ritual, the narrative of their mother's past.

The opening scene thus prepares for the eventual divergence of their paths, by briefly dramatizing apartment life before this divergence. Though Tom chooses escape, and Laura cannot, they share their family history, and our awareness of this bond at the opening of the play leads us to consider that they share the same family experiences. We do not yet know that Tom works, and Laura does not; the only reference to occupations is to Laura's typing and shorthand, and we have received no indication that Laura's business career is only wishful thinking on Amanda's part. Scene two exposes Laura's inability to pursue a career, and scene three explains Tom's frustration with his job and his life, but the play opens with the brother and sister equally engaged in tolerating their mother's dominating personality.

Scenes two and three feature dialogues between Amanda and Laura, and Amanda and Tom, respectively; Tom is not present as either narrator or character in scene two, and although Laura is present for scene three, she is almost totally silent until the end of the scene, when Tom knocks against her glass menagerie, and she cries out. Although in these two scenes we begin to see the differences between Tom and Laura, both scenes revolve around Amanda's complaints about their career choices. What does become apparent, however, is the distinction between the brother and sister that will ultimately send them to different futures, despite their shared past. In scene two, Amanda returns home and interrupts Laura washing and polishing her glass collection. When she hears Amanda ascending the fire escape, "Laura catches her breath, thrusts the bowl of ornaments away, and seats herself stiffly before the diagram of the typewriter keyboard as though it held her spellbound" (I, 151). Laura pretends to have an interest in a career, even to the point of pretending to attend business school, but she has no ambitions, no plans, no goals.

By contrast, Tom thinks of little except his plans. The typewriter that represents Laura's career failure provides Tom an escape from his warehouse job. In scene three, Amanda and Tom argue, and the stage directions tell us: "The upright typewriter now stands on the drop-leaf table, along with a wild disarray of manuscripts. The quarrel was probably precipitated by Amanda's interruption of Tom's creative labor" (I, 162). Tom dreams of a career as a writer; the lack of Laura's ambition is strongly contrasted with the artistic ambitions of Tom. Amanda berates Laura for her refusal to have a career, and interrogates Tom about the career he plans. She interrupts Laura's play, and interrupts Tom's artistic work. In Amanda's eyes, therefore, Tom's desire to find satisfying work is as dangerous to the family security as Laura's resistance to any kind of career. Being an artist is as unreliable as being a recluse.

Tom's nightly flights from the apartment stand in strong contrast to Laura's status as a "home girl." She leaves the apartment once during the play, and then it is reluctantly: she dreads an encounter with the grocer, and goes only at her mother's insistence. As she rushes out, she slips on the landing, emphasizing her lameness; her fall also signifies her inability to negotiate the world outside the apartment. Tom, on the other hand, wants adventure; while he is tied to his job at the warehouse, his only opportunity for adventure is vicarious, through the movies he attends. Although he sees his nightly wanderings as biding time, and is impatient for real adventure, we see them differently: his narrative about the movies and the magic show demonstrates his storytelling abilities, and contrasts his life with Laura's isolated one.

As a means of escape, however, Laura's withdrawal and Tom's writing are similar, and they use them in similar ways to cope with their present situation. Laura is temporarily safe from her mother's demands and from the world in general when she attends to her glass menagerie; she even uses her glass figures to explain to Jim what she has been doing since high school. Jim's interrogation of her career goals constitutes the only inquiry Laura receives since her mother gave up on that course in scene two; just making conversation, Jim inquires twice during scene seven about Laura's interests and plans. Both times Laura mentions her glass collection, explaining to Jim that it "takes up a good deal of time" (I, 220). In fact, for Laura it is a full-time job, and although Jim does not understand this, she does manage to divert his attention away from his questioning of her. As Bigsby points out:

Laura's powerlessness is symbolized by the fact that she cannot master the typewriter. Her hesitant speeches are in fact a series of withdrawals. The only language which is wholly uninfected by commerce, bitterness and disillusionment is that which she employs when describing her glass menagerie, the private language in which she addresses her own inventions. (44)

Tom uses his own form of escape, his writing, to make his life bearable. Ironically, he uses the same typewriter for his escape that represents Laura's defeat. When first describing Jim to the audience, he informs us that he was on friendly terms with Jim at work, and Jim "knew of my secret practice of retiring to a cabinet of the washroom to work on poems when business was slack in the warehouse" (I, 190). With this commentary, Tom explains his friendship with Jim, but also relates his writing practices. He is able to tolerate his life in the warehouse by fleeing to his writing whenever possible. However, his mother interrupts him when he tries to write at home, and eventually his boss ends his writing at work, for Tom tells us at the end of the play, "I was fired for writing a poem on the lid of a shoe-box" (I, 236). Losing his job proves to be the impetus for Tom's escape, and he leaves home after this, descending "the steps of this fire escape for a last time" (I, 236).

Tom's need to write, then, is stronger than his desire to protect Laura, or, for that matter, Amanda. As the opening description of Tom's character explains, he is a "poet with a job in a warehouse. His nature is not remorseless, but to escape from a trap he must act without pity" (I, 129). Not only does Tom use the experience of his family life to create art, but in order to create that art he must abandon the family. Laura's emotional and economic precariousness does not prevent Tom from taking the escape that losing his job provides, and he leaves his mother and sister to whatever fate holds for them. Tom's decision to leave is a necessary act of self-preservation, for he cannot tolerate his "two-by-four" situation; this escape is limited, however, for his closing monologue indicates that he is trapped by the memories of Laura.

From the action of this play, then, we can surmise that if the artist is not the mad person, he may contribute to the breakdown of someone he loves. While Niesen claims that in Williams's early plays the artist figure is the one who dies, and his sensitivity leads to that death, in *The Glass Menagerie* we see the pattern that Niesen identifies as that of his later plays: Tom is an "angel of death" for Laura. In this case the death is more likely a descent into madness, or at least poverty, but when Laura blows out her candles, we sense the end of her fragile existence. Williams creates a play that dramatizes that sad existence, and as the narrator of that play he distances himself from the action in order to comment on it, and provide a way in for the audience. As a character he distances himself when he descends the fire escape for the last time.

The question also becomes one of arguing whether Laura's safety or sanity is sacrificed for Tom's escape. If Williams does attempt to exorcise his personal demons by turning his family into the characters in his plays, especially in *The Glass Menagerie,* and we recognize what he is doing by its similarity to what Tom is doing, that may help us to understand the playwright. We must also consider that the statement this play makes is much more significant than a study of how one playwright deals with his sister's insanity and confinement. In an interview, Williams identified himself as an "incomplete person," claiming interest in "people that have to fight for their reason, people for whom the impact of life and experience from day to day, night to night, is difficult, people who come close to cracking" (Devlin 82). But he goes on to claim that his is not a unique perspective: "I don't think you will find many artists who aren't more or less in the same situation. Give a person an acute sensibility and you're bound to find a person who is under a good deal of torment, especially in this particular time" (82).

Tom and Laura are both sensitive people, and both suffer from the abandonment by their father, their mother's unrealistic expectations, and from the lack of opportunity offered by life in a St. Louis tenement during the Depression. The play establishes that although the brother and sister have the same background, and both seem to be the incomplete persons that Williams identifies with, they deal with their torments differently. Tom finds a creative outlet for his painful memories, and his very abandonment of Laura becomes the subject matter of the play he narrates. In the case of the characters in *The Glass Menagerie,* Pickering's theory of the "creative malady" seems to hold true, for while Tom can create, Laura is emotionally crippled by her anxieties.

If *The Glass Menagerie* represents Williams's early vision of one family's emotional instability, one of his late plays presents a variation on the theme of madness and art, and similarly focuses on a brother and sister. This play, which consumed Williams's attention during the 1970s, exists in three printed versions; it contains only two characters: both artists, both mad. This play is often compared to *The Glass Menagerie,* and R. B. Parker reports that one reviewer called it a sequel to the earlier play (523). Entitled *The Two-Character Play* at its appearance in 1967, Williams changed the name in the second version to *Out Cry;* in the third version he reverted to the original title.[4]

In a typescript version of the play dated August 1970, housed at the University of Texas, next to the typed title *The Two-Character Play,* Williams has handwritten, "or 'The Mysteries of the Incomplete.'"[5] Although this subtitle is crossed out, and was not used in any of the printed versions, it suggests that Felice and Clare represent the incomplete people he spoke of in the interview mentioned above. Of the plays in his canon, *The Two-Character Play* contains the most specific and detailed account of the artist's relation to madness. George Niesen calls the play, "Williams's most intellectually realistic statement concerning the artist's untenable and isolated position in a modern culture" (488). R. B. Parker argues that the play was Williams's attempt to grapple with the "two central and interlocked experiences of his life: his ambiguous, near-incestuous love for his schizophrenic sister, Rose; and his compulsive need for theatre as personal escape and therapy" (521). Parker's assessment of the play emphasizes the connection between the playwright's feelings about Rose and her illness, and his convictions about art as a possible guard against his own vulnerability to mental illness. This outlook on the play once more suggests that Williams saw his creativity as "passion fulfilled," and his sister's illness as "passion thwarted."

Felice and Clare, a brother and sister theatrical team, have arrived at a "state theatre of a state unknown," and the emphasis on "state" foreshadows talk of that other state, the state mental hospital (V, 313). During the play-within-the-play (also called *The Two-Character Play,* with characters named Felice and Clare), Clare mentions that the hospital where her father was treated was named "State Haven" (341). We soon learn that Felice was also confined at State Haven because as Clare tells him, "[Y]ou had allowed yourself to lose contact with all reality" (346). Felice accuses Clare of having withdrawn from reality, saying that she was at some point so disturbed that she did not know where she was. In the 1970 typescript, Clare makes another reference to State Haven cut from later versions, when the people from "Citizens Relief" leave their card under the door. Clare is relieved that "people know we're still here," to which Felice answers: "[W]here would we be but still here." Clare then replies: "They might suppose we'd been removed to—State Haven." Just after this, in a section that was also edited from the final version of the play, Clare speaks of the opal she found in an old coat pocket, which her mother said was unlucky, and Clare claims that an "unlucky birthstone might lead me into—confinement." Felice replies: "It isn't your name but my name that's in the files of State Haven, along with father's, you know." Clare indicates how closely their fates are tied, a situation that becomes more evident in the later versions, for she wonders aloud how could "your name be in the files of State Haven without some mention of mine, at least some, some—footnote of reference to me, Felice."[6] By comparing the earlier draft to the later versions, we see that Williams sought to make the charges of insanity more vague, and more shared by the two of them.

Since the inner play and its characters and discussions so closely resemble the outer frame, we assume that the situation of the inner play is based on the lives of the two actors. Felice wrote the inner play, so here is another case of the artist figure who transmutes life into art, and these lives are bound by family instability and the institutionalization of at least two family members.

At the time of the action, the actors Felice and Clare are withdrawing from reality and "going into" the play, and in this "state theatre of a state unknown" they are seeking a "state haven," some place where they can rest from the pressures of performing. At the end they remain in the theater, and this confinement reinforces the suggestion that the theater does represent an asylum. Niesen claims that the two are "struggling desperately against the tide of insanity," and in the dramatization of this struggle, Williams rejects "insanity and death as means of dealing with reality" (488). But this struggle against insanity demonstrates that even if Felice and Clare rage against madness in ways that other Williams's characters do not, the possibility still exists that insanity will engulf them. The ending of the play does not provide concrete proof that they survive the struggle with mental faculties intact.

The set provides the first indication that the two characters are mentally unbalanced, for Williams specifies in the opening stage directions that the exterior setting, the set that surrounds the play-within-the-play set, "must not only suggest the disordered images of a mind approaching collapse, but also, correspondingly, the phantasmagoria of the nightmarish world that all of us live in at present" (V, 308). With this remark Williams emphasizes his belief that the madness of his characters, and in this case the confusion and disorder of the set, correspond to the world of the audience: he is not dramatizing merely a private, individual madness but the collective madness of the modern world. The stage directions then introduce Felice, and in the initial description of him we see the depiction of the mad artist, for he is defined as a "playwright, as well as player, but you would be likely to take him for a poet with sensibilities perhaps a bit deranged" (V, 309).

In the first two versions of the play, Clare tries to explain why others might consider the siblings insane, for she tells her brother, "[Y]ou know that artists put so much into being artists, I mean into their work, that they've got very little left over for acting like other people, their behavior is bound to seem peculiar" (TTCP, 13). Although this remark is cut from the final edition, the spirit of the remark remains, with its idea that Felice and Clare are perceived as deranged because of their preoccupation with their art.

Clare's first appearance identifies her as abnormal. Before she enters, Felice worries about keeping her from "getting too panicky to give a good performance," adding that she is "not easy to fool in spite of her—condition" (V, 310). The stage directions then inform us that "her condition when she appears is 'stoned,'" which is a component of her instability, but her reliance on pills and drugs seems to be a by-product of her reaction to the family's mental problems, and not the sole source of her nervousness. After making her entrance, Clare, who dangles a tiara from her fingers, "gives a slight startled laugh when she notices it, shrugs, and sets it crookedly on her somewhat disheveled and streaked blonde head" (V, 311). The tiara associates Clare with other disturbed female protagonists, most notably Blanche, who also wears what Stanley calls her "crazy crown," a rhinestone tiara, just before the rape scene. Since the tiara is not a prop that Clare would need in the performance she is about to give, its presence seems significant for its representation of Clare's "craziness."

The identification of Clare with demented women who take on royal personas continues a few pages later, when she sees a throne-chair onstage and calls out, "My God, old Aquitaine Eleanor's throne! I'm going to usurp it a moment—," sitting on the chair "as if to hold court" (V, 314). Throughout this stage business, Felice and Clare accuse each other of a variety of sins, displaying hostility toward each other, as well as the conviction that each knows what is best for the other. Felice suggests that Clare take an "upper," to which she responds that she never drops an "upper" before the performance; Clare suggests that Felice take his codeine for the migraine he complains about, to which he replies that he has "never found that narcotics improve a performance" (V, 314). The scene sets up a dynamic rarely found in Williams's plays about madness, for usually the mad person stands in strong contrast to the others in the play, those who appear sane. Here, however, the only two characters in the work are both unstable, and each accuses the other of mentally unbalanced behavior.

Since the play is set in a theater, and the characters are both actors (and Felice is a playwright), the world of the play is charged by an atmosphere of make-believe, with the focus on the unreality of the theater. This atmosphere is reinforced by the lack of clear boundaries between the outer play and the play-within-the-play, for the more the two become indistinguishable, the more the audience or reader feels unbalanced. The effect is to immerse the audience in the confusion and disorientation that the characters themselves express.

What we do have in commentary from the world outside damns Felice and Clare, and serves to inform us that they are both right about each other, and neither possesses the rationality to condemn the other's behavior. Although the rest of the theater company has left them before the play opens, a cablegram seems to represent the judgment of the rest of the world. When Clare makes repeated demands to know why the stage is deserted except for them, Felice shows her the cablegram, which explains that the company left because "Your sister and you are— *insane!*—Having received no pay since—" (321). In the 1970 typescript, when Clare reads the cablegram, she assumes that Felice has given them the impression that he is insane, by all his "obsessive rewrites." Naturally, the company would be offended by it, and "come to the conclusion that you were not just an eccentric artist but *un peu derange*. And you'd fallen into a habit of shouting out at rehearsals 'Mad, I'm going mad!' So finally they took your word for it, cher."[7] Felice responds that the cablegram said that they were both insane, not just him, and this enrages her, for she does not want to be implicated in causing the desertion of the company.

At this point in the play, we discover that Felice and Clare have no place to go: not only have they been deserted by their company, but they did not check into a hotel when they arrived at this latest "state unknown." When Clare speaks of escape, of going to the hotel to collapse, Felice reminds her that no hotel haven is available to them. This predicament leads them to begin the performance of the play-within-the-play, and although Clare resists, Felice convinces her that it is their only option. In their move into the inner play, we come to discover more about the two, for we are able to piece together aspects of their lives that led them to the abandoned theater in their current state.

The characters in the inner play are confined in their family home, just as the actors Felice and Clare are confined in the theater. The characters in the inner play are isolated from the community in which they live, partly because of their eccentric behavior, but primarily because their father, who was mentally disturbed, killed his wife and himself and left his children to bear the burden of his act. The 1970 typescript gives more detail about this incident: when Felice rambles on about the giant sunflower, Clare yells, "Shut up or I'll call State Haven." This is followed by the information, in parentheses, that this is the "precise threat which had precipitated the 'accident' in the house.'"[8] Thus we know that not only was their father insane, but that the threat of confinement drove him to murder and suicide.

Since Felice too has been confined in State Haven, and since both brother and sister fear confinement, they might be driven to kill themselves; this prefigures the situation at the conclusion of the play. They cannot face the neighborhood's curiosity and scorn; they hide themselves away, thus convincing the townspeople that they are insane. Clare speaks on the phone to a minister, and in trying to obtain his help, she explains the circumstances that led them to hide from the community. In a direct parallel to the cablegram the other Felice and Clare received from their company, Clare tells the Reverend that accusations about her and her brother's mental instability come through the mail, "anomalous letters of obscenities are sent us, and in *The Press Scimitar*—sly allusions to us as the deranged children of a father who was a false mystic" (V, 337-38).

Thus the judgment of insanity comes from outside as well as from within, for while each sibling accuses the other of irrational behavior, the community of the play-within-the-play and the company of the outer play judge both Felice and Clare to be insane. Niesen compares *The Two-Character Play* to Beckett's plays, and claims that "Godotlike outer worlds are associated with both the frame and the play, but Clare and Felice can function in neither outer world. They are confined to their roles as actors and artists" (Niesen 489). The nature of their confinement is indeed significant to the understanding of the intersection between madness and art, for here we can establish whether, in Williams's world-view, art or madness, or some combination of the two, provides a viable escape from the harshness of the world.

Felice and Clare argue over their artistry, each one attempting to establish a position of dominance over the other. Their first disagreement concerns who is better equipped to handle the press, even after Felice informs Clare that they "don't have to face the press before this evening's performance" (V, 312). Each accuses the other of alienating the press with theoretical ramblings, Clare's political in nature, and Felice's artistic. Next they argue about whether or not to cancel the performance, and Clare insists that Felice envies her superior acting skills, accusing him of not forgiving her "for my Cleopatra notices. Ran into columns of extravagance and your Anthonys were condensed as canned milk" (V, 317).

If Clare successfully establishes control by flaunting her greater skill as an actor, Felice retakes the position of power by focusing on his role as the playwright, and he decides what play they will perform. Clare then emphasizes his method of control by asking her brother, "Are you going to throw new speeches at me tonight?" (V, 318). Felice replies that "there'll have to be a lot of improvisation" (V, 318). This mention of improvisation indicates that the creative struggle will become part of the inner play, for the two are free to insert lines that may force the other's hand, or call for spontaneous (and therefore unguarded) response.

Clare counters with her own plan for altering her brother's creative work, informing him that since he has not instituted the cuts she asked for, she will make them herself. Felice protests, insisting: "Where my work is concerned—," implying that she may not tamper with his art. Clare holds her ground, maintaining that total theater "is going to be total collaboration on this occasion" (V, 324). This collaboration becomes a central factor in the outcome of Williams's play, for as they struggle over the direction that the action of the inner play takes, we see that this struggle will also determine what will happen to the "real" Felice and Clare, as well as what will happen to the characters of the inner play.

Clare's insistence that she have some control over the actions of the inner play sets up a situation in which both characters are creators, and this is a rare situation in a Williams play. *The Two-Character Play* dramatizes the conflicts between a twosome who are equally matched in both mental condition and possession of artistic sensibility. The play provides a unique perspective on madness and the artist, for most of

Williams's plays that deal with these subjects contrast characters of different sensibilities. Here the conflicts exist between two characters of equal strength and weakness, who see in each other their own faults and vulnerabilities.

Williams takes considerable care to present Felice and Clare as equals, not opposites. Besides the judgment of the acting company that they are both insane, the two speak of various others who have compared them and found them to be alike. Clare tells Felice of a doctor who proclaimed that the two were the bravest people he knew, to which Clare replied, "Why, that's absurd, my brother and I are terrified of our shadows" (V, 311). Later, within the inner play, brother and sister speak of leaving their house, and when Felice encourages Clare to go out, she insists that she would "never dream of going out without you in your— disturbed—*condition.*" Felice counters with, "And *you* in *yours*" (V, 336).

When Clare calls the Reverend, she speaks of herself and Felice as a pair, emphasizing their similar condition, in that the townspeople think of them both as deranged. In Act Two, their plan is to go to Grossman's Market to secure provisions, and Felice speaks of making the errand together, entering "Grossman's Market today like a pair of—" (V, 343). Finally, when they emerge from the inner play, and speak of leaving the theater, Felice encourages them to look for accommodations at the hotel across the street. He tells her that "we'll enter in such grand style that we'll need no reservations" (V, 361). When Felice goes to check the theater door, he leaves Clare alone on the stage, and she responds in panic, calling to him to "Hurry back! I'm alone here!" (V, 361). Felice and Clare cannot be separated, for if they are, they both agree that they would end up permanently alone, "locked in separate buildings and marched out at different hours" (V, 357). Clare rejects this fate for them because of "what a long, long way we've traveled together, too long, now, for separation" (V, 357). If this play is a kind of sequel to *The Glass Menagerie,* this brother and sister do not end up separated, as Tom and Laura do. Felice and Clare both choose art as an outlet for their anxieties, but their theater work does not relieve them of their torment, even if it provides a temporary means of survival. Their companionship, however, offers them comfort.

Felice and Clare provide the clearest example of Williams's protagonists who openly speak of the fear of confinement. When the characters in the inner play argue about Clare's calling the Reverend for assistance, Felice insists on the danger of telling their problems to a "man who'll think it his Christian duty to have us *confined* in—" (V, 338). Clare reacts violently to his use of this word, and she exclaims that the "word is not in the—" (V, 338). We do not know, but might guess that she would have finished her sentence with the "play," and such an ending would suggest that Felice's use of that word forces Clare out of concentration, and out of character. When she speaks, it is as the actor Clare, who is also afraid of confinement. Felice calls "confined" a prohibited word, saying that when a word is prohibited, "its silence increases its size" (V, 338).

Williams recalls this moment of the play in his *Memoirs*, when he notes that confinement "has always been the greatest dread of my life: that can be seen in my play *Out Cry*" (*Memoirs* 233). As Sy Kahn observes, for Williams "the theater has been the agency for freedom, both personal and artistic, but, as he discovered, and as the entrapped Felice and Clare symbolize, it can also be a prison" (51). Kahn argues that *Out Cry* expresses "Williams's ambivalences toward the theater, which at once was his *raison d'etre,* his arena of artistic expression and freedom, but whose circle is a tightening noose . . . the theater is a deceptively gilded cage for a bird freely to sing the paradoxical songs of its entrapped existence" (52).

Talk of the prohibited word so upsets the two actors that it brings them out of the inner play, and the act ends with a physical struggle between them; Felice picks up a pillow and puts it over Clare's mouth. Their struggle and the break in the play indicates that their attempts to use the play as a means of avoiding their fate, their isolation from the world and their eventual confinement in the theater, only works temporarily until their struggle once more becomes the central issue. This conclusion of the first act foreshadows the conclusion of the entire play, when the two become locked in a possibly fatal struggle over whether or not to use the gun. This aspect of struggle is essential to the play because it illustrates the similarity of the two characters' situations and mental condition. Since they are both unbalanced, the struggle for dominance is equal, and never decided clearly. The siblings argue over the issues that we are exploring in this chapter: insanity and art.

In Williams's earlier plays that feature characters who are called insane, or who are artists, this is not the case. In *The Glass Menagerie,* Tom's struggle to escape and his decision to choose his art over his sister's well-being is never contested by Laura herself. The *Two-Character Play* is often considered, along with the *Night of the Iguana,* the most optimistic of Williams's plays, because it ends with a rejection of the double suicide that Felice and Clare seem to feel is their only escape. Their dogged insistence to continue living suggests that despite their indefinite imprisonment in the locked theater, they can face whatever happens rather than escape it through death. Again the 1970 typescript provides more information about Williams's view of the ending, for he toyed with a number of epigraphs before deciding on "A garden enclosed is my sister." Written on the title page of the manuscript, and then crossed out, is a quotation he attributes to Hemingway, "Man can be destroyed but not defeated."[9] This quotation suggests the ambiguity of the ending of the play, that though the pair are destroyed by their past, and by their current circumstances, life has not defeated them, and they continue to carry on in whatever small way they can. Part of their strength comes from their ability to continue with their art, even without an audience, and without a clear ending for the play they perform. Their creative talents thus provide an outlet for their panic and their instability, but this is not a conventional happy ending by any means.

The conclusion of the play is as ambiguous as that of *The Glass Menagerie*. In that play we do not know what happens to Laura, and do not know what happens to Tom; likewise, we cannot be sure that Felice and Clare will continue to find comfort in acting. We do not know if Tom's memory play serves to expunge his demons, and we do not know if Felice and Clare will continue to embrace life and reject the end the revolver would bring. The author's notes to the 1970 typescript states that "two desperately gallant but hopelessly deviant beings, find themselves, in the end, with no escape but self destruction, which fails them too."[10]

The difference lies, of course, in the sheer number of survivors in each play: in *The Glass Menagerie,* Tom tells Laura to blow out her candles, and from his final narration we know that he is alone. *The Two-Character Play* ends with the embrace of the principals; not only are the brother and sister alike in temperament, they are devoted to each other, and show throughout the play that they would never actually abandon one another. If Williams makes a statement in the two plays about how artistry can protect one from the ravages of madness, and particularly from institutionalization, those artists are more fortunate who have a companion in the battle.

Tom Wingfield escapes his family situation relatively intact, but he wanders alone, "more faithful" to Laura and his past than he would wish. Felice and Clare are also haunted by their tragic family memories, and they have transmuted those memories into art, but they have each other to perform them with: they are able to comfort each other when the performance is over. Williams's statement in this play is that art and madness do interconnect in his artist figures, for the sensitivity necessary to produce creative works predisposes the artist to the ravages of insanity (along with such related problems as alcoholism and drug addiction).

The inability or lack of opportunity to transmute suffering into art can induce madness, and the sensitive figure who does not or cannot create is perhaps even more vulnerable. Laura is the ultimate example of this; in the case of Laura and Tom, they share the same family experience, they both suffer from their imperfect family life, but Tom does not go insane, he writes a play. Felice and Clare both become artists to escape from their tragic family experience, but they struggle with insanity, and recognize the inherited instability in each other. Nonetheless, they do not end up in mental hospitals, or as suicides: they continue to perform their art as a means of survival. They choose not to commit suicide, even though the play-within-the-play allows for this as one possible ending; however, they are trapped in a theater in a northern state in winter, and they have no idea when they might be able to leave.

To say that this ending is more optimistic than those of other Williams plays is only to say that the two survive at the end, not that they are happy or productive members of society. As Niesen claims: "[T]he gun of the abnormality of family insanity is apparently pointed at them, rendering them powerless to leave the house, the stage, or the theater"; however, Niesen also insists that Felice and Clare "endure for the time of the play. They survive. They make a feeble attempt at creating art" (Niesen 492). What makes this survival particularly poignant is the fact that they face their struggles together, and they end the play in a moment of communion: "They reach out their hands to one another, and the light lingers a moment on their hands lifting toward each other. As they slowly embrace, there is total dark in which: THE CURTAIN FALLS" (370).

Because Williams was a master of paradox, as we see in most of his best plays, his interest and examination of the artist and madness are extremely enlightening, for it is a relationship steeped in paradox. Despite the arguments of such theorists as Albert Rothenberg, who attempt to discredit stereotypes of the mad genius, we cannot simply categorize those with creative powers as either sane or not. Williams's artist figures are complex, and although his works indicate that the artistic sensibility is often vulnerable, it would seem that for Williams, art can provide an escape from annihilation as readily as it provides a passageway to it. As in the case of Williams's women characters, we must be cautious not to leap to a single or one-sided conclusion. In the character of Tom Wingfield, Williams embodies the artist who achieves escape through his work, although this escape does not preclude painful memories and even an obsession with the past. Felice and Clare face madness because of their family history, and they use art to endure.

In *Clothes for a Summer Hotel,* Williams has Zelda Fitzgerald make a specific statement about madness and the artist, claiming that life is all "an arranged pattern of—submission to what's been prescribed for us unless we escape into madness or into acts of creation" (*Clothes* 71). In the two plays I have examined in this chapter, Williams dramatizes this view, and also shows that they are not mutually exclusive situations. In *The Two-Character Play,* the artists do resemble the eccentric genius of the stereotype, and in this respect Williams upholds the romantic notion that art is born of great emotional suffering, the kind of emotional trauma that might as easily cause mental breakdown. At the same time, the plays examined here show that art can be a means of survival, and that although that survival is tenuous, those who have no artistic outlet are more likely to end up annihilated, like Laura. If suffering and emotional trauma lead through struggle to the creation of art, they might just as easily cause insanity. Zelda's words emphasize how closely connected are the two outcomes, madness and acts of creation.

5

Broken Worlds: Conclusion

Nowadays is, indeed, lit by lightning, a plague has
stricken the moths, and Blanche has been put away.
—Williams's *Memoirs*

In *Dimensions of the Modern Novel,* Theodore Ziolkowski's final
chapter proposes that the German fiction of the 1960s is a "land of insanity, abnormality and absurdity without parallel . . . a veritable bedlam of
madmen" (332-35). Expanding his claim to encompass other forms of literature, he cites the number of German theatrical successes set in asylums, among them *The Physicists* and *Marat/Sade.* Ziolkowski claims
that insanity "represents the final stage of a process: it is the ultimate
intensification of the role of the outsider who is rejected by society or
who himself rejects society—alternatives which in the final analysis produce the same effect" (335). Although Foucault places madness within
the context of his study of the Age of Reason, he argues that madness
claims thematic importance much earlier: "Indeed, from the fifteenth
century on, the face of madness has haunted the imagination of Western
man" (15). At this time, according to Foucault: "[T]he mockery of madness replaces death and its solemnity" (15). He sees death and madness
as linked, as part of the same anxiety: "What is in question is still the
nothingness of existence, but this nothingness is no longer considered an
external, final term, both threat and conclusion; it is experienced from
within as the continuous and constant form of existence" (16).

In his drama, Tennessee Williams implies that society, threatened by
madness, reacts by suppressing behavior that appears menacing; his
plays suggest that individual freedom and originality are sacrificed to
maintain the community's illusions about its normalcy. Not that Williams was the first playwright to dramatize madness: from the furious
frenzies of Ajax or Agave to the twisted truths of Ophelia, Lear, and various mad fools, the stage has borne witness to centuries of mad ravings.
While O'Neill preceded Williams in bringing the subject to the modern
American stage, and other playwrights have dramatized madness,
Williams's dramas distinctively portray his mad characters with a combi-

101

nation of brutal honesty and tenderness. Perhaps more than any other
modern playwright, he creates these characters with sympathy, while not
succumbing to the Romantic view that the mad hold the secrets to all
knowledge and understanding. Although their sensibilities may be finer,
and more highly developed, they are deeply troubled by their emotional
problems and fare worse than their coarser counterparts. Sometimes the
nervous types may seem superior to those around them, but more often
they are destroyed and "put away." Women are especially susceptible to
such a fate; only slightly less so are artists, unless they establish an outlet
for their emotional turmoil in creative work.

Madness has a definite affiliation with other subjects Williams
chose for his dramas. Not only does his family history reveal that such a
topic arises from Williams's own experience, but throughout his years of
writing he himself gravitated toward the most shocking, the most unmentionable of human actions. Donald Spoto cites Henry Popkin's
remark in the *Tulane Drama Review:* "Williams now seems to be in a
sort of race with himself, surpassing homosexuality with cannibalism,
cannibalism with castration, devising new and greater shocks in each
succeeding play" (258). But a difference exists between a subject such as
cannibalism, a taboo rarely transgressed in Western culture, and the
madness which he portrays in many of his plays. Although the mad have
been hidden away, in the attic and in the asylum, their anxieties are bred
in circumstances and events that mirror our own. To see a mad person on
stage may be shocking, but madness exists within the boundaries of
human experience; the disintegration of the mind rivals death as one of
the most fearful fates. Williams chooses to propose as equally frightening the idea that judgments about insanity may be based on subjective
anxieties, and that objective diagnosis is an illusion.

By dramatizing the plight of the madman and madwoman, people too
fragile to survive the tortures of memory or the brutality of others, Williams
established a name for himself in modern literature as a champion of the
outsider. These "weak and divided people" are removed from the main-
stream when their behavior upsets the tenuous balance that the other characters have achieved in their lives; although the community strains towards
normalcy, it is easily upset by the appearance of the one deemed mad. As
close study of the individual plays has shown us, the mad person usually
insists on verbalizing the corruption hidden beneath the facade of normalcy
and rationality. For these revelations, the punishment also provides a solu-
tion: confinement disciplines the transgressors, and silences them.

My examination of the mad characters in Williams's plays has
attempted to show that despite their ultimate restraint, these characters
mark the world they enter and upset; they make an impression on the

world that they pass through on their way to the asylum. Stanley tells Blanche that she has "left nothing here but spilt talcum and old empty perfume bottles," but those of us who have witnessed the play know that Blanche has transformed more than the apartment decor when she passes through Elysian Fields. She has transformed us, at least momentarily, into a society capable of sympathy for its broken victims. William Kleb says that Blanche's legacy is her "Otherness," now planted in Stanley because of the rape, which now "stands between Stella and Stanley at the end of the Williams's play" (40). Perhaps just the opposite occurs for the audience: we see her "Otherness" as Sameness. Because Williams took such care with his portrayal of Blanche, she becomes more than an interfering in-law, a pathetic drunk, a promiscuous schoolteacher masquerading as a lady. She becomes a woman whose loss of control touches us because we see through her experience how close the edge is, how quickly and unexpectedly our own sanity could come into question.

Blanche may be the most memorable of Williams's characters, but others hold our interest and earn our sympathy. All three Wingfields capture our attention, and we see in them the frailties of small people with desires thwarted by life or luck. The troubled members of this family feel acutely the discrepancies between their lives as they imagine them and as they actually are. Lucretia Collins has allowed the memory of a girlhood romantic attachment to shut her off completely from any meaningful human contact. Her loneliness and isolation mirror the plight of many in today's cities. Violet Venable, struggling to convince herself of the purity of her son's life, seeks to ensure her own life's usefulness, terrified that Sebastian's sordid death renders her own existence a "trail of debris." Her tactics are ruthless, but we can understand her need to create a version of her life that demonstrates her importance. Catharine's terror that the truth may sentence her to a mindless life, lobotomized and institutionalized, encapsulates our common fear that if we are punished for what we believe, our freedom diminishes.

These characters display less than attractive qualities as well, prompting us to accept the full range of human behavior, asking us to consider the view of humanity that Hannah Jelkes espouses: "Nothing human disgusts me unless it's unkind, violent" (IV, 363-64). Perhaps this statement illuminates the most insistent statement of Williams's drama: that the bravest stand requires a clear, unflinching outlook combined with a measure of empathy. Among the array of characters Williams created, Hannah very nearly represents the only embodiment of this combination, an indication of how rarely strength and sensitivity mesh. As much as Williams insists on the superiority of such a combination, so does he consistently demonstrate its rarity through his dramas.

Notes

Chapter 1

1. Tennessee Williams, Letter to Rev. and Mrs. W. E. Dakin, 13 Oct. 1939, Humanities Research Center, U of Texas, Austin.

2. Tennessee Williams, Letter to Edwina and C. C. Williams, 21 Mar. 1939, Humanities Research Center, U of Texas, Austin.

3. Tennessee Williams, Letter to Edwina and C. C. Williams, 5 Aug. 1928, Humanities Research Center, U of Texas, Austin.

4. Tennessee Williams, Postcard to Edwina Williams, 4 Apr. 1938, Humanities Research Center, U of Texas, Austin.

5. Audrey Wood, Letter to Tennessee Williams, 7 July 1943, Humanities Research Center, U of Texas, Austin.

6. Rose Williams, Letter to Tom Williams, 1 Jan. 1937, Humanities Research Center, U of Texas, Austin.

7. Tennessee Williams, Letter to Edwina Williams, May 1943, Humanities Research Center, U of Texas, Austin.

8. Tennessee Williams, Letter to Audrey Wood, Dec. 1939, Humanities Research Center, U of Texas, Austin.

9. Tennessee Williams, Letter to Walter Dakin, 3 June 1952, Humanities Research Center, U of Texas, Austin.

10. Anon, "The Angel of the Odd," *Time Magazine*, 9 Mar. 1962: 53.

11. All quotations are taken from Michel Foucault, *Madness and Civilization: A History of Insanity in the Age of Reason*, trans. Richard Howard (New York: Vintage, 1988). Originally published in French as *Histoire de la Folie*, by Librairie Plon, 1961, and in the United States by Pantheon, 1965.

12. I discuss this further and in specific connection to two of the plays in the chapter on language, for in both *Streetcar* and *Suddenly Last Summer* the confinement of Blanche and Catharine, respectively, rests on the stories that these women tell.

13. Many people who are not insane are confined to mental hospitals; most often, these are people who cannot provide for their own needs, because of some physical or mental handicap. Such institutionalization carries a social stigma, nonetheless. Many consider all inmates of an asylum "crazy," not distinguishing between those who have been clinically diagnosed as insane, and those who suffer from blindness or alcoholism.

14. The distinction is made by the society of the play, however, between sexual behavior within a relationship sanctioned by society, and activities outside those boundaries. Stella and Blanche of *Streetcar* both have strong sex drives; Stella seeks satisfaction within her marriage, and her pregnancy represents the result of her sanctioned sexual relationship with Stanley. Blanche's desire for younger men and "intimacies with strangers" falls outside the approved parameters.

15. Tennessee Williams, "The Night of the Iguana," typescript (hereafter ts.) Humanities Research Center, U of Texas, Austin, undated. All typescripts will be referenced by notes, as most are not paginated. Whenever possible I refer to the version published in *The Theatre of Tennessee Williams*.

16. Williams, "Iguana," ts., undated.

17. Dates listed after play title are of first performance.

18. Tennessee Williams, *A Streetcar Named Desire, The Theatre of Tennessee Williams*, 8 vols. to date, (New York: New Directions, 1971-1992). Unless otherwise indicated, all quotations from the works will be from this edition, and will be indicated by notations in the text with volume number and page number.

19. Tennessee Williams, "Summer and Smoke," ts., Humanities Research Center, U of Texas, Austin, November 1946: 8.

20. In chapter 3, I explore this difference in depth by focusing on the particular qualities of the female madwoman in Williams's plays. Social and economic conditions particular to women seem to contribute to their vulnerability for institutionalization.

21. Williams, "Iguana," ts., undated.

22. Williams, "Iguana," ts., undated.

23. Williams, "Iguana," ts., undated.

24. In O'Neill's early sea plays, such as *Bound East for Cardiff*, the set significantly minimized the available space to portray the experience of sailors in the hull, in order to focus on the narrowness of their lives. *The Hairy Ape*'s set directions specify that the ceiling of the ship's forecastle crushes down upon the men's heads. In the original production of *Desire under the Elms*, the actors crouch in tiny rooms overshadowed by the suffocating elm trees that represent the repressive atmosphere of the Cabot home. For a photograph of this set, see Christopher Bigsby, *A Critical Introduction to Twentieth-Century American Drama*, 3 vols. (Cambridge: Cambridge UP, 1982), Vol. 1: 65. Bigsby says this about O'Neill's plays: "[T]he space available for character to form, for language to coalesce, and for social visions to expand, is minimal. The dominant image is one of constriction" (63).

25. Carol Rosen, *Plays of Impasse: Contemporary Drama Set In Confining Institutions* (Princeton: Princeton UP, 1983). The asylum plays she chooses

to examine are Peter Weiss's *Marat/Sade* (1964), Friedrich Durrenmatt's *The Physicists* (1962), and David Storey's *Home* (1970).

26. Tennessee Williams, "Stairs to the Roof," Undated ts., Humanities Research Center, U of Texas, Austin. The foreword is dated Dec. 1941.

27. Shirle Duggan, review, "Los Angeles Examiner," ts., Humanities Research Center, U of Austin, Texas.

28. Tennessee Williams, quoted by Ruth Loring, review, Humanities Research Center, U of Austin, Texas.

29. Goffman defines total institutions as those institutions in our society whose "encompassing or total character is symbolized by the barrier to social intercourse with the outside and to departure that is often built right into the physical plant, such as locked doors, high walls, barbed wire, cliffs, water, forests, or moors." Although Goffman's primary focus is on mental asylums, he supplements this discussion with plentiful examples of treatment in prisons, concentration camps, military establishments, and even boarding schools.

30. Williams, ts., undated.

31. Tennessee Williams, *The Two-Character Play*, ts., Humanities Research Center, U of Texas, Austin, undated: 12.

32. Williams, ts.: 23.

33. Brooks Atkinson, "Garden District," rev. of *Suddenly Last Summer* and *Something Unspoken, New York Times,* 19 Jan. 1958.

34. Harold Clurman, "Nightlight and Daylight," article on acting, unidentified publication, on file in Humanities Research Center, U of Austin, Texas, Feb. 1948.

35. Seymour Peck, "Williams and 'The Iguana,'" rev. of *The Night of the Iguana, New York Times*, 24 Dec. 1961.

Chapter 2

1. Most of the articles I quote in this section either predate or exclude plays written after *The Night of the Iguana*, that is, after 1961.

2. See W. J. Cash, *The Mind of the South* (Garden City: Doubleday Anchor, 1954). Jones uses Cash's theory of the mythically cavalier Old South to explain the motivations of Williams's women who cannot face the reality of modern life, escaping through illusion into a "legendary world that never really was." These former southern aristocrats steadily degenerate as they withdraw from the world, becoming increasingly alienated from it.

3. Chesler's book book shares the title with Ripa's study of nineteenth century France. Chesler, an American psychologist and feminist, centers her discussion on contemporary women and finds many of the same attitudes and assumptions intact in the 1970s in the United States. The striking similarities demonstrate that women have faced prejudice about their emotional stability in this century no less than in previously "unenlightened" times.

4. Although Blanche DuBois is widowed, she calls herself an "old maid schoolteacher."

5. When Williams saw the production he decided that Jessica Tandy, who played the lead, would play Blanche in the production of *Streetcar* later that year.

6. Yannick Ripa suggests that in the popular imagination madness was often seen as a "punishment better than death, which would be too much. It was a half-death, the death of the mind" (2).

7. This "date" represents the culmination of all the points of conflict between the two, both as individuals, and as representatives of opposing social groups.

8. Durant da Ponte, for example, holds that the climax indicates that the lobotomy is performed on Catharine, although the play gives no clear evidence to support this (da Ponte 15); Nancy M. Tischler and others suggest that Violet is the insane one, who "goes mad when the merciful veil is stripped from the unendurable truth"; see *Tennessee Williams: Rebellious Puritan* (New York, 1965).

9. Williams uses various sources for the details of the Fitzgeralds' relationship, including Nancy's Milford's 1970 biography, *Zelda*, and Hemingway's 1964 *A Movable Feast*. Thomas Adler discusses in detail Williams's use of the Milford book; see Thomas P. Adler, "When Clothes Supplant Memories: Tennessee Williams' *Clothes for a Summer Hotel*," *Southern Literary Journal* 19.2 (1987): 5-19.

10. Williams had his own rather unsuccessful stint working in Hollywood as a screenwriter. In 1943, Audrey Wood negotiated for Williams a six-month contract as a screenwriter, where he was assigned to write a screenplay for Lana Turner. He could not reconcile working on what he called a "celluloid brassiere" for the star, and was eventually suspended from his contract for refusing to work on assigned material. Given this course of events, one can appreciate Scott's assertion in *Clothes* that he is "selling his talent" in order to secure a steady income for his family.

Chapter 3

1. We do not know whether Mitch believes Blanche about the rape; it is possible that the truth of it would only confirm his decision about Blanche, that she is "not clean enough to bring in the house" with his mother. His presence at the second poker game, even though he makes an ineffective move to protect Blanche from the Matron's attempts to subdue her, shows that he goes along the path of least resistance.

2. Tennessee Williams, *Suddenly Last Summer*, ts., Humanities Research Center, U of Texas, Austin, undated. All quotations from *Suddenly* are from this manuscript, unless otherwise noted in the text.

3. Williams, *Suddenly Last Summer,* ts.

4. Williams, *Suddenly Last Summer,* ts.

5. Richard Watts, Jr., "Two Dramas by Tennessee Williams," rev. of *Suddenly Last Summer* and *Something Unspoken* by Tennessee Williams, *New York Post,* 8 Jan. 1958: 64.

6. Tennessee Williams, *The Two-Character Play,* ts., Humanities Research Center, Austin, 1970: Author's notes.

7. Williams, ts., 1970.

8. David Savron argues that *In the Bar of a Tokyo Hotel* has been misunderstood by its critics, and that the play marks an important development in Williams' writings: "an insistent and radical fragmentation of discourse, character, and plot that is far more aggressive and overt than that which marks even the most surrealistic of his earlier plays." See David Savron, *Communists, Cowboys, and Queers: The Politics of Masculinity in the Work of Arthur Miller and Tennessee Williams* (Minneapolis: U of Minnesota P, 1992): 135.

Chapter 4

1. Donald Spoto speaks of Williams's fear of madness a number of times in his biography of the playwright, saying that during the sixties, Williams considered his "artistic, physical, and emotional condition hopeless; his plays acknowledged that, even as their creation was a brave bid to prevent his total collapse" (Spoto 295). Spoto also quotes Williams as claiming to have "a touch of schizophrenia in me and in order to avoid madness I have to work" (337).

2. Also see Tennessee Williams, *The Two-Character Play* (New York: New Directions, 1969) 57. All other notations of this edition will be marked as *TTCP*, with the page number. In this, the first published version of a play that also focuses on a brother and sister, and specifically mentions insanity, the brother Felice warns his sister: "Don't you know your behavior, if it goes on like this, will get the two of us hauled by force out of the house and put like two wild animals in separate, locked, barred cages in what's called a zoo or a zoological garden—publicly naked for the grinning to stare at?" This description of an asylum as a zoo indicates that Williams may have had something similar in mind when he associates Laura with the zoo and the glass house. Both images signal confinement and observation, the two main components of an asylum.

3. Letter from Williams to Audrey Wood, undated, Humanities Research Center, U of Texas, Austin.

4. While my discussion will not dwell on the differences among the three versions (since this has been the topic of numerous other essays), I will refer primarily to the last published version, assuming that this is the version Williams considered the "final version." However, I will also include some references to my topic that appear only in one of the earlier versions, as evidence of Williams's preoccupation with madness.

5. Tennessee Williams, "The Two-Character Play," ts., Humanities Research Center, U of Texas, Austin, 1970.

6. Williams, ts., 1970.

7. Williams, ts., 1970.

8. Williams, ts., 1970.

9. Williams, ts., 1970.

10. Williams, ts., 1970.

Selected Bibliography

Primary Works

Collection

The Theatre of Tennessee Williams. 8 volumes. New York: New Directions, 1971-1992.

Battle of Angels. New York: New Directions, 1945.

27 Wagons Full of Cotton and Other One-Act Plays. Norfolk: New Directions, 1945; London: Grey Walls, 1947. Contains *27 Wagons Full of Cotton, The Purification; The Lady of Larkspur Lotion, The Last of My Solid Gold Watches, Portrait of a Madonna, Auto-Da-Fe, Lord Byron's Love Letters, The Strangest Kind of Romance, The Long Goodbye, Hello from Bertha, This Property Is Condemned, Talk to Me Like the Rain and Let Me Listen . . .*, and *Something Unspoken.*

A Streetcar Named Desire. New York: New Directions, 1947.

You Touched Me! With Donald Windham. New York: French, 1947.

American Blues: Five Short Plays. New York: Dramatists Play Service, 1948. Contains *Moony's Kid Don't Cry, The Dark Room, The Case of the Crushed Petunias, The Long Stay Cut Short,* or *The Unsatisfactory Supper,* and *Ten Blocks on the Camino Real.*

One Arm and Other Stories. New York: New Directions, 1948.

Summer and Smoke. New York: New Directions, 1948.

The Roman Spring of Mrs. Stone. New York: New Directions, 1950.

I Rise in Flame, Cried the Phoenix. New York: New Directions, 1951.

The Rose Tattoo. New York: New Directions, 1951.

Camino Real. Norfolk: New Directions, 1953.

Hard Candy: A Book of Stories. New York: New Directions, 1954.

Cat on a Hot Tin Roof. New York: New Directions, 1955. Rev. ed. New York: New Directions, 1975.

Baby Doll. New York: New Directions, 1956.

Orpheus Descending. London: Secker & Warburg, 1958. *Orpheus Descending, with Battle of Angels.* New York: New Directions, 1958.

Suddenly Last Summer. New York: New Directions, 1958.

Garden District. London: Secker & Warburg, 1959.

Sweet Bird of Youth. New York: New Directions, 1959.

Period of Adjustment. New York: New Directions, 1960.

Three Players of a Summer Game and Other Stories. London: Secker & Warburg, 1960.

The Night of the Iguana. New York: New Directions, 1962.

The Eccentricities of a Nightingale and Summer and Smoke. New York: New Directions, 1964.

Grand. New York: House of Books, 1964.

The Milk Train Doesn't Stop Here Anymore. New York: New Directions, 1964.

In the Winter of Cities: Poems. Norfolk: New Directions, 1964.

The Knightly Quest: A Novella and Four Short Stories. New York: New Directions, 1967. New York: New Directions, 1967. Revised and enlarged as *The Knightly Quest: A Novella and Twelve Short Stories.* London: Secker & Warburg, 1968.

Kingdom of Earth (The Seven Descents of Myrtle). New York: New Directions, 1968. Rev. ed. New York: Dramatists Play Service, 1969.

Dragon Country: A Book of Plays. New York: New Directions, 1969. Contains *In the Bar of a Tokyo Hotel, I Rise in Flame, Cried the Phoenix, The Mutilated, I Can't Imagine Tomorrow, Confessional, The Frosted Glass Coffin, The Gnadiges Fraulein,* and *A Perfect Analysis Given by a Parrot.*

In the Bar of a Tokyo Hotel. New York: Dramatists Play Service, 1969.

The Two-Character Play. New York: New Directions, 1969.

Small Craft Warnings. New York: New Directions, 1972.

Out Cry. New York: New Directions, 1973.

Eight Mortal Ladies Possessed: A Book of Stories. New York: New Directions, 1974.

Memoirs. Garden City: Doubleday, 1975.

Moise and the World of Reason. New York: Simon & Schuster, 1975.

Androgyne, Mon Amour: Poems. New York: New Directions, 1977.

Where I Live: Selected Essays. Ed. Christine R. Day and Bob Woods. New York: New Directions, 1978.

Vieux Carre. New York: New Directions, 1979.

A Lovely Sunday for Creve Coeur. New York: New Directions, 1980.

Clothes for a Summer Hotel: A Ghost Play. New York: New Directions, 1983.

Stopped Rocking and Other Screenplays. New York: New Directions, 1984. Contains *Stopped Rocking, All Gaul Is Divided, The Loss of a Teardrop Diamond,* and *One Arm.*

The Red Devil Battery Sign. New York: New Directions, 1988.

Something Cloudy, Something Clear. New York: New Directions, 1995.

Collected Letters and Interviews

Conversations with Tennessee Williams. Ed. Albert J. Devlin. Jackson: UP of Mississippi, 1986.

Five O'Clock Angel: Letters of Tennessee Williams to Maria St. Just, 1948-1982. With commentary by Maria St. Just. New York: Knopf, 1990.

Tennessee Williams's Letters to Donald Windham 1940-1965. Ed. Donald Windham. New York: Holt, 1977.

Secondary Works

Adler, Thomas P. *American Drama 1940-1960: A Critical History*. New York: Twayne, 1994.

——. *A Streetcar Named Desire: The Moth and the Lantern*. Boston: Hall, 1990.

Al-Issa, Ishan. *The Psychopathology of Women*. Englewood Cliffs: Prentice-Hall, 1980.

Atkinson, Brooks. "Garden District." *New York Times* 19 Jan. 1958.

Bentley, Eric. *In Search of Theatre*. New York: Knopf, 1953.

Berman, Jeffrey. *The Talking Cure: Literary Representations of Psychoanalysis*. New York: New York UP, 1985.

Bigsby, C. W. E. *A Critical Introduction to Twentieth-Century American Drama, volume 2: Williams, Miller, Albee*. Cambridge: Cambridge UP, 1984.

——. *Modern American Drama, 1945-1990*. Cambridge: Cambridge UP, 1992.

Blackwell, Louise. "Tennessee Williams and the Predicament of Women." *Tennessee Williams: A Collection of Critical Essays*. Ed. Stephen S. Stanton. Englewood Cliffs: Prentice Hall, 1977. 100-06.

Bloom, Harold, ed. *The Glass Menagerie: Modern Critical Interpretations*. New York: Chelsea, 1988.

——, ed. *A Streetcar Named Desire. Modern Critical Interpretations*. New York: Chelsea, 1988.

——, ed. *Tennessee Williams: Modern Critical Views*. New York: Chelsea, 1987.

Boxill, Roger. *Tennessee Williams*. London: Macmillan, 1987.

Bynum, W. F., Roy Porter, and Michael Shepherd, eds. *The Anatomy of Madness: Essays in the History of Psychiatry*. 2 vols. New York: Tavistock, 1985.

Chesler, Phyllis. *Women and Madness*. New York: Avon, 1972.

Clark, Robert A., M.D. *Mental Illness in Perspective: History and Schools of Thought*. Pacific Grove, CA: Boxwood, 1973.

Cohn, Ruby. *Dialogue in American Drama*. Bloomington: Indiana UP, 1971.

——. "Late Tennessee Williams." *Modern Drama* 27.1 (1984): 336-44.

——. "Tributes to Wives." *The Tennessee Williams Review*. 4.1 (1983): 12-17.

Da Ponte, Durant. "Williams' Feminine Characters." *Tennessee Studies in Literature* 10 (1965): 7-26.

Davis, Joseph K. "Landscapes of the Dislocated Mind in Williams' *The Glass Menagerie*." *Tennessee Williams: A Tribute*. Ed. Jac Tharpe. Jackson: UP of Mississippi, 1977. 192-206.

Devlin, Albert J. *Conversations with Tennessee Williams*. Jackson: UP of Mississippi, 1986.

Donahue, Francis. *The Dramatic World of Tennessee Williams*. New York: Ungar, 1964.

Falk, Signi L. *Tennessee Williams*. Boston: Twayne, 1961. Rev. 1978.

Fedder, Norman J. *The Influence of D.H. Lawrence on Tennessee Williams*. The Hague: Mouton, 1966.

Feder, Lillian. *Madness in Literature*. Princeton: Princeton UP, 1980.

Felman, Shoshana. *Writing and Madness*. Trans. Martha Noel Evans and the author. Ithaca: Cornell UP, 1985.

Foucault, Michel. *Madness and Civilization: A History of Insanity in the Age of Reason*. Trans. Richard Howard. 1965. New York: Vintage, 1973.

——. *The Order of Things: An Archaeology of the Human Sciences*. New York: Vintage, 1973.

Franks, Violet, and Esther D. Rothblum, eds. *The Stereotyping of Women: Its Effects on Mental Health*. New York: Springer, 1983.

Gilbert, Sandra M., and Susan Gubar. *The Madwoman in the Attic: The Woman Writer and the 19th Century Literary Imagination*. New Haven: Yale UP, 1979.

Gilman, Sander L. *Difference and Pathology: Stereotypes of Sexuality, Race, and Madness*. Ithaca: Cornell UP, 1985.

——. *Disease and Representation: Images of Illness from Madness to AIDS*. Ithaca: Cornell UP, 1988.

——. *Seeing the Insane*. New York: Wiley, 1982.

Goffman, Erving. *Asylums: Essays on the Social Situation of Mental Patients and Other Inmates*. Garden City: Doubleday Anchor, 1961.

Griffin, Alice. *Understanding Tennessee Williams*. Columbia: U of South Carolina P, 1995.

Gunn, Drewey Wayne. *Tennessee Williams: A Bibliography*. 1980. Metuchen: Scarecrow, 1991.

Hauptmann, Robert. *The Pathological Vision: Jean Genet, Louis-Ferdinand Celine, and Tennessee Williams*. New York: Peter Lang, 1984.

Hayman, Ronald. *Tennessee Williams: Everyone Else Is an Audience*. New Haven: Yale UP, 1993.

Haynal, Andre. *Depression and Creativity*. New York: International UP, 1985.

Heilman, Robert Bechtold. *The Iceman, the Arsonist, and the Troubled Agent: Tragedy and Melodrama on the Modern Stage*. Seattle: U of Washington P, 1973.

Hirsch, Foster. *A Portrait of the Artist: The Plays of Tennessee Williams*. Port Washington: Kennikat, 1979.

Howell, Elizabeth, and Marjorie Bayes, eds. *Women and Mental Health*. New York. Basic, 1981.

Ingram, Allan. *The Madhouse of Language: Writing and Reading Madness in the Eighteenth Century*. London: Routledge, 1991.

Jackson, Esther Merle. *The Broken World of Tennessee Williams*. Madison: U of Wisconsin P, 1965.

——. "The Synthetic Myth." *Tennessee Williams*. Ed. Harold Bloom. New York: Chelsea, 1987. 23-42.

Jones, Robert Emmet. "Sexual Roles in the Works of Tennessee Williams." *Tennessee Williams: A Tribute*. Ed. Jac Tharpe. Jackson: U of Mississippi P, 1977. 545-57.

——. "Tennessee Williams' Early Heroines." *Modern Drama* 2 (1959): 211-19.

Kahn, Sy M. "Listening to *Out Cry:* Bird of Paradox in a Gilded Cage." *New Essays on American Drama*. Ed. Gilbert Debusscher and Henry I. Schvey. Atlanta: Rodopi, 1989. 41-62.

Kaplan, Bert, ed. *The Inner World of Mental Illness*. New York: Harper, 1964.

Kaplan, Cora. *Sea Changes: Essays on Culture and Feminism*. London: Verso, 1986.

Kataria, Gulshan Rai. *The Faces of Eve: A Study of Tennessee Williams's Heroines*. New Delhi: Sterling Publishers Private Limited, 1992.

King, Thomas L. "Irony and Distance in *The Glass Menagerie*." Rpt. in *Tennessee Williams*. Ed. Harold Bloom. New York: Chelsea, 1987. 85-94.

Kleb, William. "Marginalia: *Streetcar*, Williams, and Foucault." *Confronting Tennessee Williams's* A Streetcar Named Desire*: Essays in Critical Pluralism*. Ed. Philip C. Kolin. Westport: Greenwood, 1993. 27-43.

Laing, R. D. *The Divided Self*. New York: Pantheon, 1960.

——. *The Politics of Experience*. New York: Pantheon, 1967.

——, and A. Esterson. *Sanity, Madness and the Family*. London: Tavistock, 1964.

Leverich, Lyle. *Tom: The Unknown Tennessee Williams*. New York: Crown, 1995.

Londre, Felicia Hardison. *Tennessee Williams*. New York: Ungar, 1979.

Martin, Philip W. *Mad Women in Romantic Writing*. New York: St. Martin's, 1987.

McCann, John S. *The Critical Reputation of Tennessee Williams: A Reference Guide*. Boston: Hall, 1983.

McGlinn, Jeanne M. "Tennessee Williams' Women: Illusion and Reality, Sexuality and Love." *Tennessee Williams: A Tribute*. Ed. Jac Tharpe. Jackson: UP of Mississippi, 1977. 510-24.

Melman, Lindy. "A Captive Maid: Blanche Dubois in *A Streetcar Named Desire*." *Dutch Quarterly Review of Anglo-American Letters*. 16.2 (1986): 125-44.

Miller, Jordan Y., ed. *Twentieth Century Interpretations of A Streetcar Named Desire*. Englewood Cliffs: Prentice-Hall, 1971.

Mitchell, Juliet. *Psychoanalysis and Feminism*. New York: Pantheon, 1974.

Morrow, Laura, and Edward Morrow. "The Ontological Potentialities of Antichaos and Adaptation in *A Streetcar Named Desire*." *Confronting Tennessee Williams's* A Streetcar Named Desire: *Essays in Critical Pluralism*. Ed. Philip C. Kolin. Westport: Greenwood, 1993. 59-70.

Murphy, Brenda. *Tennessee Williams and Elia Kazan: A Collaboration in the Theatre*. Cambridge: Cambridge UP, 1992.

Nelson, Benjamin. *Tennessee Williams: The Man and His Work*. New York: Oblensky, 1961.

Niesen, George. "The Artist Against the Reality in the Plays of Tennessee Williams." *Tennessee Williams: A Tribute*. Ed. Jac Tharpe. Jackson: UP of Mississippi, 1977. 463-93.

Pagan, Nicholas. *Rethinking Literary Biography: A Postmodern Approach to Tennessee Williams*. Rutherford, NJ: Fairleigh Dickinson UP, 1993.

Parker, R. B. "The Circle Closed: A Psychological Reading of *The Glass Menagerie* and *The Two-Character Play*." *Modern Drama* 28.4 1985: 517-34.

Peck, Seymour. "Williams and the 'Iguana.'" *New York Times* 24 Dec. 1961.

Perry, John Weir. *Roots of Renewal in Myth and Madness*. San Francisco: Jossey-Bass, 1976.

Phillips, Gene D. *The Films of Tennessee Williams*. East Brunswick: Associated UP, 1980.

Pickering, George. *Creative Malady*. London: Allen & Unwin, 1974.

Porter, Roy. *Mind-Forged Manacles: A History of Madness in England from the Restoration to the Regency*. Cambridge: Harvard UP, 1987.

——. *A Social History of Madness: The World Through the Eyes of the Insane*. 1987. New York: Dutton, 1989.

Porter, Thomas E. *Myth and Modern American Drama*. Detroit: Wayne State UP, 1969.

Presley, Delma E. *The Glass Menagerie: An American Memory*. Boston: Hall, 1990.

Rader, Dotson. *Tennessee: Cry of the Heart*. New York: Plume, 1985.

Redmond, James, ed. *Madness in Drama*. Cambridge: Cambridge UP, 1993.

Rieger, Branimir M., ed. *Dionysus in Literature: Essays on Literary Madness*. Bowling Green, OH: Bowling Green State University Popular Press, 1994.

Ripa, Yannick. *Women and Madness: The Incarceration of Women in Nineteenth-Century France*. Trans. Catherine du Peloux Menage. Cambridge, UK: Polity, 1990.

Robinson, Marc. *The Other American Drama*. Cambridge: Cambridge UP, 1994.

Rosen, Carol. *Plays of Impasse: Contemporary Drama Set in Confining Institutions*. Princeton: Princeton UP, 1983.

Rothenberg, Albert, M.D. *Creativity and Madness: New Findings and Old Stereotypes*. Baltimore: John Hopkins UP, 1990.

Sahu, Dharanidhar. *Cats on a Hot Tin Roof: A Study of Alienated Characters in the Major Plays of Tennessee Williams*. Delhi: Academic Foundation, 1990.

Sass, Louis A. *Madness and Modernism: Insanity in the Light of Modern Art, Literature, and Thought.* New York: Harper Collins, 1992.

Savran, David. *Communists, Cowboys, and Queers: The Politics of Masculinity in the Work of Arthur Miller and Tennessee Williams.* Minneapolis: U of Minnesota P, 1992.

Schlueter, June. *Dramatic Closure: Reading the End.* Rutherford: Fairleigh Dickinson UP, 1995.

——, ed. *Feminist Rereadings of Modern American Drama.* Rutherford: Fairleigh Dickinson, 1989.

Shaland, Irene. *Tennessee Williams on the Soviet Stage.* Lanham, MD: UP of America, 1987.

Showalter, Elaine. *The Female Malady: Women, Madness, and English Culture, 1830-1980.* New York: Pantheon, 1985.

Sievers, W. David. *Freud on Broadway: A History of Psychoanalysis and the American Drama.* New York: Cooper Square, 1955.

Simon, Bennett, M.D. *Mind and Madness in Ancient Greece: The Classical Roots of Modern Psychiatry.* Ithaca: Cornell UP, 1978.

Smith, Bruce. *Costly Performances. Tennessee Williams: The Last Stage.* New York: Paragon, 1990.

Spoto, Donald. *The Kindness of Strangers: The Life of Tennessee Williams.* Boston: Little, Brown, 1985. Rpt., Ballantine, 1986.

Stanton, Stephen S., ed. *Tennessee Williams: A Collection of Critical Essays.* Englewood Cliffs: Prentice-Hall, 1977.

Steen, Mike. *A Look at Tennessee Williams.* New York: Hawthorn, 1969.

Szasz, Thomas S., M.D. *Law, Liberty, and Psychiatry: An Inquiry into the Social Uses of Mental Health Practices.* 1963. Syracuse: Syracuse UP, 1989.

——. *The Manufacture of Madness: A Comparative Study of the Inquisition and the Mental Health Movement.* New York: Harper, 1970.

——. "The Myth of Mental Illness." *Ideology and Insanity: Essays on the Psychiatric Dehumanization of Man.* Garden City: Doubleday, 1970.

Tharpe, Jac, ed. *Tennessee Williams: A Tribute.* Jackson: UP of Mississippi, 1977.

Thompson, Judith J. *Tennessee Williams's Plays: Memory, Myth, and Symbol.* New York: Lang, 1987.

Tischler, Nancy M. "A Gallery of Witches." *Tennessee Williams: A Tribute.* Ed. Jac Tharpe. Jackson: UP of Mississippi, 1977. 494-509.

——. *Tennessee Williams: Rebellious Puritan.* New York: Citadel, 1963.

Van Antwerp, Margaret A., and Sally Johns, eds. *Dictionary of Literary Biography Documentary Series.* vol. 4. *Tennessee Williams.* Detroit: Gale, 1984.

Vernon, John. *The Garden and the Map: Schizophrenia in Twentieth-Century Literature and Culture.* Chicago: U of Illinois P, 1973.

Vlasopolos, Anca. "Authorizing History: Victimization in *A Streetcar Named Desire*." *Feminist Rereadings of Modern American Drama*. Ed. June Schlueter. Rutherford: Fairleigh Dickinson UP, 1989. 149-70.

Watts, Richard, Jr. "The Magic of Tennessee Williams." *New York Post* 19 Jan. 1958: 21.

Weales, Gerald. *Tennessee Williams*. Minneapolis: U of Minnesota P, 1965.

Weissman, Philip. "A Trio of Tennessee Williams' Heroines: The Psychology of Prostitution." *Creativity in the Theater: A Psychoanalytic Study*. New York: Basic, 1965. 173-89.

Whitworth, Walter. "Uta Hagen Is Superb in *A Streetcar Named Desire*." *Indianapolis News* 7 Oct. 1948: 17.

Williams, Dakin, and Shepherd Mead. *Tennessee Williams: An Intimate Biography*. New York: Arbor, 1983.

Williams, Edwina Dakin, as told to Lucy Freeman. *Remember Me to Tom*. New York: Putnam, 1963.

Windham, Donald. *Lost Friendships: A Memoir of Truman Capote, Tennessee Williams, and Others*. New York: Morrow, 1987.

Yacowar, Maurice. *Tennessee Williams and Film*. New York: Ungar, 1977.

Index

119